Carcinoid Tumors

Carcinoid Tumors
A Clinicopathologic Study

Charles Marks

M.D., M.S., Ph.D., F.R.C.P., F.R.C.S., F.A.C.S.,
F.C.C.P., F.A.C.C.

Professor of Surgery, Louisiana State University
  School of Medicine
Attending Surgeon, Charity Hospital, Veterans Administration
  Hospital, Touro Infirmary, and Hotel Dieu Hospital
Consultant Cardiovascular Surgeon, East Jefferson
  and Methodist Hospital, New Orleans, Louisiana
  Former Hunterian Professor
Royal College of Surgeons of England

G. K. HALL & CO.
Boston, Massachusetts

CARCINOID TUMORS

Marks, Charles

Copyright © 1979
G. K. Hall & Co.
Medical Publications Division
70 Lincoln St.
Boston, Massachusetts 02111

Library of Congress Catalog No. 78-11390
ISBN 0-8161-2141-9

Includes bibliographical references and index.
1. Carcinoid.   2. Alimentary canal—Tumors.
3. Bronchi—Tumors.   I. Title.   [DNLM: 1. Carcinoid
tumor.   WI435 M346c]
RC280.A4M37   616.9'94

The authors and publisher have worked to ensure that all information in this book concerning drug dosages, schedules, and routes of administration is accurate at the time of publication. As medical research and practice advance, however, therapeutic standards may change. For this reason, and because human and mechanical errors will sometimes occur, we recommend that our readers consult the *PDR* or a manufacturer's product information sheet prior to prescribing or administering any drug discussed in this volume.

With dedication to my wife Joyce and to my sons Malcolm, Peter, Ian, and Anthony

Foreword

The quest to solve the mysteries of cancer has led to an accumulation of comprehensive information about the natures of many tumors. Yet scientific information about carcinoid tumors, a unique, infrequent type of neoplasm, is limited. The objective of the detailed study in this monograph is to elucidate the occurrence, the course of events, and the therapeutic responses of these tumors.

Skilled as an internist, a surgeon, and a scientist, Dr. Marks has thoroughly analyzed an unprecedented series of cases from our teaching institutions. The clinical, pathological, and therapeutic information should be of inestimable value as the definitive reference for clinicians, pathologists, and oncologists on the subject of carcinoid tumors.

Paul F. Larson, M.D.
Dean
Louisiana State University
School of Medicine
New Orleans, Louisiana
October 31, 1978

Preface

In 1978, English-speaking surgeons celebrated the 250th anniversary of the birth of John Hunter. Hunter was a key force in creating the scientific background of surgery and in fusing laboratory investigation with clinical study. It was he who wrote to Edward Jenner, "Why think? Why not try the experiment?" The product of the Hunterian tradition—the modern surgeon—has well been described as "a physician who is condemned to operate." The operation itself is merely one aspect of a surgeon's total involvement with a patient. The surgeon must also consider the pathology of the patient's disease, the existing investigations, and the patient's psychological and physiological responses to both the illness and surgery.

In this monograph, Charles Marks, with his wide background of surgical training in South Africa, the United Kingdom, and the U.S.A., demonstrates that he is a worthy Hunterian. He takes an uncommon, fascinating tumor and, drawing upon his broad clinical experience with 172 patients who have this condition at the Charity and the Veterans Administration Hospitals in New Orleans, paints a broad canvas for us. We are taken through the historical background of the disease, its biochemical peculiarities and markers, its pathology (from naked eye appearance to electron microscopy), and its relation to other cancers and multiple endocrine abnormalities. Careful consideration of pathology provides a useful guide to both treatment and prognosis. The encouraging results of the treatment of liver metastases and the development of specific drugs to combat the malign effects of the carcinoid syndrome follow logically from Dr. Marks' deep understanding of the pathological and biochemical effects of carcinoid tumors.

Other physicians, whose experience of this disease is confined to

Preface

the occasional cases which occur in their own practice, will be grateful to Dr. Marks who so happily blends art and science in this beautiful monograph.

Harold Ellis, M.D., M.Ch., F.R.C.S.
Professor of Surgery
Westminster Medical School, University
   of London
London, 1978

Contents

Chapter 1

Introduction

From 1948 to 1971, 172 patients with carcinoid tumors were seen at Charity Hospital and Veterans Administration Hospital in New Orleans. One hundred thirty-five patients presented with carcinoids of the gastrointestinal tract. Thirteen patients represented a distinct group of carcinoid-islet cell tumors of the duodenum that justify distinct categorization, and 24 patients had bronchial adenomas of the carcinoid type.

In order to determine the natural history of carcinoid tumors at specific sites, the carcinoids were grouped according to location and mode of discovery. Table 1 compares our experience with the collected cases in the world. We found no patients with carcinoids of the esophagus, gall bladder, Meckel's diverticulum, pancreas, or ovary.

Attention was directed to the data of 106 clinical patients with gastrointestinal carcinoids. The clinical features, mode of diagnosis, treatment, pathologic features, and the presence or absence of coexisting disease were analyzed. Twenty-nine carcinoid tumors of the gastrointestinal tract represented incidental findings at autopsy and had produced no clinical symptoms. These cases were included only when pathologic features or the presence of coexisting disease were considered (Table 2).

The carcinoid tumors of the gastrointestinal tract were categorized according to size under one of three headings:

1. less than 1 cm
2. 1 to 2 cm
3. 2 cm or larger

Carcinoid Tumors

Table 1. Carcinoid Tumors

Site	Collected Cases	Present Series
Esophagus	1	0
Bronchus	1% of Primary Lung Tumors	24
Stomach	98	10
Duodenum	135	25 (12 conventional) (13 carcinoid-islet cells)
Jejunoileum	1,032	37
Meckel's diverticulum	46	0
Appendix	1,686	29
Colon	94	10
Rectum	706	37
Pancreas	2	0
Biliary tract	10	0
Ovary	34	0

Table 2. Location and Method of Discovery

Location	Clincial	Autopsy	Total
Bronchus	20	4	24
Stomach	8	2	10
Duodenum	21	4	25
Jejunoileum	18	19	37
Colon	8	2	10
Rectum	37	0	37
Appendix	27	2	29
Total	139	33	172

The appropriate size of tumors was obtained from the description recorded by clinicians, surgeons, or pathologists. The definition of size appeared important and a search was made for correlation between tumor size, the presence of symptoms, and extent of the disease process. Follow-up information was available in 102 of the 106 clinical patients and was provided by outpatient clinic reports or tumor registries (Morgan, Marks and Hearn, 1974).

Analysis of the 13 patients with carcinoid-islet cell tumors of the duodenum draws heavily on the previously published reports of this series of cases. Significant clinical differences justify consideration of this group within a separate and distinctive category.

The 24 patients with bronchial carcinoid tumors represented 86% of all the bronchial adenomas seen during this time; 3 (11%) were cylindromatous and 1 (3%) was a mucoepidermoid tumor. During this period 4553 cases of primary bronchogenic tumors were seen at these institutions. Bronchial adenoma represented 0.6% of all primary lung tumors. This study of the natural history of bronchial carcinoids reviews clinical symptoms and signs as well as radiologic and bronchoscopic findings. The presence of associated disease and the relationship of bronchial carcinoids to the polyendocrine syndrome is reviewed in the light of our experience.

If bronchial carcinoids are excluded, the total world collected series of carcinoid tumors accounts for less than 4000 cases (Table 1). Comparison between our institutional experience and the world experience is summarized in Figure 1.

The carcinoid tumor is generally considered to be a neoplasm that contains argentaffin cells derived from the Kulchitsky cells of the small intestine. Although tumors arising from sites other than the small intestines have been reported with clinical and biochemical findings previously associated with this classical definition of carcinoid tumors, they lacked argentaffin characteristics.

The classification of carcinoid tumors based on their origin from differing embryologic divisions of the primitive gut delineates as follows (see Table 3):

1. differences in histologic structure
2. variations in histochemical reaction
3. association with the carcinoid syndrome

3

CARCINOID TUMORS
Site Distribution

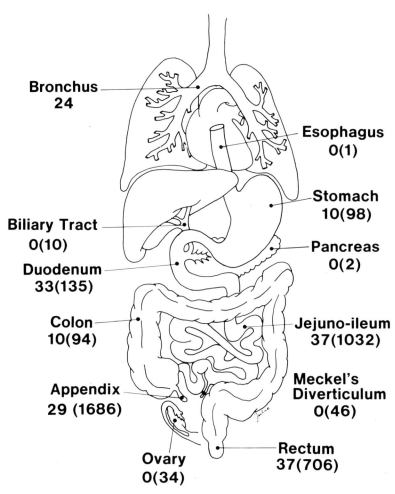

Bronchus
24

Esophagus
0(1)

Stomach
10(98)

Biliary Tract
0(10)

Pancreas
0(2)

Duodenum
33(135)

Colon
10(94)

Jejuno-ileum
37(1032)

Appendix
29 (1686)

Meckel's
Diverticulum
0(46)

Rectum
37(706)

Ovary
0(34)

Fig. 1: Site distribution of carcinoid tumors. Figures in parentheses represent collected world series.

Table 3. Correlative Features of Carcinoid Tumors Based on Embryologic Derivation.
Predominant Features of Carcinoids in Relation to Primary Growth Sites

	Foregut	Midgut	Hindgut
Histology Silver imp.	B type argyrophil and nonreactive	A type argentaffin	Mixed type nonreactive
Biochemistry	5 HTP, tumor Serum, urine 5 HT, urine Histamine Serum, urine 5 HIAA, urine	5 HT, tumor Serum, urine 5 HIAA, urine	
Secretory Granules EM	Round, variably dense	Pleomorphic uniformly dense	Round, variably dense
Clinical	Bright red, Geographic Pattern	Mixed cyanosis Erythema	

NOTE: 135 carcinoid tumors of gastrointestinal tract L.S.U. affiliated hospitals.

4. changes in serum and urinary components of the tryptophan cycle
5. differences in the probability of metastases

Review of the Literature

Merling reported a case of primary carcinoma of the appendix in 1838; his description of the lesion is generally accepted as the first reference to a carcinoid of this organ. Carcinoma of the appendix is a rare condition, and it is now generally known that carcinoids represent the commonest tumors of the appendix. In 1867 Langhans described the first documented case of an ileal carcinoid, describing it as a "drusenpolyp." In 1882 Beger reported details of an adenocarcinoma of the appendix, thus providing microscopic information that, retrospectively, indicates that the lesion was a carcinoid.

In 1888 Lubarsch described two autopsy cases and complemented the gross study of the intestinal tumors with histologic examination. The first case demonstrated two small tumors situated in the ileum. In the second case, he described six small tumors in the lower ileum of a 52-year-old male. He described each of these tumors as small nodules of whitish tissue situated in the submucosa and involving the muscularis. The lesions were composed of nests and strands of epithelial cells arranged in a fashion quite unlike the conventional cylindrical arrangement of intestinal mucosal cells. Serial sections through the tumors demonstrated that these epithelial nests and strands were connected with the crypts of Lieberkühn. He considered that these tumors represented an outgrowth from the glands of the intestinal mucosa. The cells were arranged in a pseudoglandular pattern with small spaces within the cell nests arranged radially around an apparent glandular lumen. The presence of pink-staining amorphous material in the clear spaces led Lubarsch to conclude that these spaces were not lumina but probably vacuoles caused by cell necrosis. Although Lubarsch described his cases as primary carcinomata of the ileum, it is apparent that he provided a classic description of carcinoids of the ileum characterized by:

1. Multiplicity of the tumors.
2. Absence of a true glandular structure.
3. The tumors were of epithelial origin and traceable to the crypts of Lieberkühn.
4. Absence of metastases.

The apparent benignity of these lesions was questioned by Ransom who, in 1890, described a patient with a small tumor in the ileum that had invaded beyond the peritoneal covering into the mesentery. The microscopic appearance resembled that described by Lubarsch, except that there were multiple secondary tumors in the liver identical in histologic structure with the tumor in the ileum. Ransom stressed that the mesenteric lymph nodes were free of metastases. As there was no other primary neoplasm anywhere in the body, it was apparent that these lesions could metastasize.

This malignant propensity was confirmed by Notthaft who, in 1896, described a patient in whom three tumors were found in the jejunum with invasion by one of the tumors into the mesentery. Nests of tumor cells were also present in the adjacent lymph nodes.

In 1904 Krompecher described a patient with six small tumors in the distal ileum. There was no invasion of the intestinal wall and no lymph node metastases. Serial section studies confirmed a direct connection between the crypts of Lieberkühn and the tumor cell nests in the submucosa.

Uncertainty regarding the nature of this tumor persisted until 1907 when Oberndorfer presented the results of his study of six cases of multiple tumors of the small intestine at the meeting of the German Pathological Society in Dresden. At this time he came to the conclusion that these tumors were:

1. Usually multiple.
2. Circumscribed with little tendency to infiltrate the surrounding tissues.
3. Nonmetastasizing.
4. Slow growing, never attaining large size.
5. Harmless and benign.
6. Situated in the submucosa, and sometimes extending into the mucosa.
7. The muscularis mucosa is always intact.
8. The stroma always consists of smooth muscle derived from the muscularis mucosa.
9. The cells are largely undifferentiated masses that may demonstrate glandular forms.

As the characteristics were those of a nonmalignant entity, he suggested that though these lesions had the appearance of carcinoma they were benign lesions. He considered their resemblance to carcinoma as attributable to their origin as an embryologic malformation and suggested they be named "Karzinoide." Despite several fundamental erroneous inferences made by Oberndorfer, these conclusions stand as a classic landmark in our understanding of the carcinoid tumor.

Oberndorfer's postulate that the tumors were probably embryologic malformations was based upon the views of Trappe (1907) who thought that carcinoids and adenomyomas represented pancreatic rests and that the carcinoid was the poorly developed example of such rests. These rests occur frequently in the gastrointestinal tract. In his view the two conditions had a common origin with the development of subtle morphologic differences. The adenomyoma, considered to be a more highly developed outgrowth of these rests, was thought to provide differentiated glandular tissue associated with well-formed ducts that communicated with the crypts of Lieberkühn. The carcinoid, on the other hand, was thought to represent a lower order of development from these pancreatic rests in which the epithelial cells did not differentiate but remained in a disorganized state with a greater capacity for growth.

In 1910 Huebschmann, in a discussion regarding carcinoids of the appendix, suggested that the yellow coloration classically associated with carcinoids was due to their origin from the yellow chromaffin cells of the intestinal mucosa. Gosset and Masson (1914) noted that the silver staining of granules in the tumor was identical with that in the chromaffin cell, thereby providing proof that the tumor indeed arose from the chromaffin cell and providing a basis for naming the tumor Argentaffinoma.

Burkhardt (1909) previously studied a group of carcinoids of the intestine and provided criteria of differentiation from adenomyomata and from accessory pancreatic formations by:

1. the absence of a muscular stroma
2. the absence of pancreatic acini
3. the failure to identify ducts or ductules
4. the identifiable connection of the tumor nests with the crypts of Lieberkühn
5. the invasive nature of the tumor
6. the production of metastases

In defining the lesion as a true tumor, Burkhardt was of the opinion that it was derived from the basal cells. He concluded that, as the tumors were derived directly from the intestinal epithelium and were composed of undifferentiated cells that manifested a low degree of malignancy as well as possessing a hyaline fibrillar stroma, they were basal cell cancers. As late as 1904 Krompecher concluded, on the basis of his histologic studies, that the carcinoid was a basal cell cancer analagous to that of skin cancer and was derived from two possible sources:

1. the basal cells of the crypts of Lieberkühn
2. from displaced cylindrical epithelial rests

Toenniessen (1910) considered the carcinoids to be the result of the development of submucous rests. He thought that they represented glands of internal secretion, and he emphasized the similarity between the cell nests of carcinoids and the islands of Langerhans. Saltykow (1912) thought that carcinoids were derived from pancreatic rests with the development of the islets only. He contrasted this with adenomyomata that consisted of glandular structures associated with ducts and a supporting connective tissue framework and that was representative of the other pancreatic components. In a discussion of the subject before the German Pathological Society, Oberndorfer emphasized the fact that the carcinoid cell cytoplasm yielded a definite chrome reaction and that it contained many doubly refractile substances.

Gosset and Masson (1914) studied the chromaffin cells of the intestinal tract using the silver impregnation technique. They indicated that these cells occurred in the depths of the crypts of Lieberkühn throughout the gastrointestinal tract. These cells were situated between the cylindrical cells of the mucosa. In some cases they extended from the basement membrane to the lumen; in others, there was no contact with the lumen. They emphasized that the argentaffin granules were always demonstrable in these cells, being located between the basement membrane and the nucleus. They attributed the vacuoles in the cytoplasm to secretory products of the granules and suggested that the cells represented an endocrine gland of entodermic origin similar to the islets of Langerhans. They concluded that the argentaffin cells could proliferate and form a conglomerate mass of tissue.

The cells that compose the carcinoid tumor were noted to be identical with the cells of the chromaffin tissue of the paraganglia which contain argentaffin granules. The only difference between these two structures was the larger quantity of lipids contained within the tumor. They also noted a microchemical similarity between the carcinoid cells and the cells of the adrenal medulla. As a result of the microchemical and morphologic similarity of the chromaffin cells of the crypts of Lieberkühn and the carcinoid tumors, Gosset and Masson concluded that these tumors were of endocrine origin and should be considered as endocrine tumors.

Hasegawa (1923) and Danisch (1924) confirmed the findings of Gosset and Masson and agreed that the carcinoids could arise either directly from the Kulchitsky cells of the crypts of Lieberkühn or from epithelial rests. Forbus (1925) concluded that they arose from the chromaffin cells of the crypts of Lieberkühn and thus should be categorized as endocrine tumors or tumors of the paraganglionic system.

These small, dark-staining argentaffin cells were first noted by Heidenhain in 1870 as small, dark-staining round cells in the stomach wall of animals exposed to potassium dichromate. He erroneously considered them to be precursors of the gastric parietal cells and did not demonstrate the granular appearance that was described later. In 1888, Paneth described cells in the crypts of the fundic gastric glands containing cytoplasmic granules. In 1897 Kulchitsky identified the granular cells in the crypts of Lieberkühn and noted that the granules increased when a high protein diet was administered and decreased if starvation was instituted.

These argentaffin cells are distributed throughout the gastrointestinal tract of the entire vertebrate kingdom. They are most profuse in the terminal ileum and appendix and rather sparse in other parts of the intestinal tract. The cells have also been noted to exist in the biliary tract as well as in Meckel's diverticulum. The cells occur singly in close relationship to the basement membrane, although, on occasion, they have been found to exist in pairs. They are generally situated between the mucous and columnar cells of the intestinal epithelium. The basal granules are not found in the unfixed state of the tissues but are precipitated by the chemical interaction between the formalin fixative and its contained secretion. The secretion was later demonstrated as 5-hydroxytryptamine (serotonin).

Although the cells were thought to be derived from the embryologic entodermal gut lining, the studies of Masson and Gosset strongly suggested that they arose from the ectoderm derived from the neural crest. These neural crest cells migrate to the intestine as they do to the adrenal medulla, the glomus jugulare, the posterior pituitary, the carotid body, and sympathetic nerve terminal processes. These cells have been identified in the large gut of the 12-week human fetus where they often exist in large numbers, appearing in groups of four to five cells clumped closely together. As this migration occurs long before the cells develop their silver reaction potential, failure to differentiate may determine the differences between the argentaffin and argyrophil reactions, as well as the failure to take up silver stains at all.

Carcinoid Tumors and Apud Cells

Apud cells have a demonstrable capacity for amine precursor uptake and decarboxylation and have been found scattered throughout the gut, bronchus, pituitary, thyroid, pancreatic islets, and adrenal gland, after having migrated from a neural crest ectodermal origin. Tumors arising from these cells have been classified as apudomas and may secrete polypeptide hormones. Hormone-producing carcinoid tumors may exist alone or may be associated with hormone-producing tumors of endocrine organs. The polyhormonal disorders are representative of multiple endocrine neoplasia, which often occur in categoric association.

Type I. Involvement of the pancreatic islets, adrenal cortex, parathyroid glands and pituitary.

Type II. Medullary thyroid carcinoma and pheochromocytoma (Sipple's disease) with chief cell parathyroid hyperplasia or adenoma.

Type III. A syndrome characterized by mucosal neuromas, medullary thyroid carcinoma, and/or pheochromocytoma in association with bumpy lips.

Chapter 2

Fundamental Effects of Carcinoid Tumors

Tryptophan is universally distributed in living species. This amino acid is utilized predominantly in the synthesis of protein as well as in the production of niacin. One percent of the tryptophan is utilized in the production of 5-hydroxytryptamine, which is found in most living beings including vertebrates and flowering plants. In 1868, Ludwig and Schmidt noted the presence of a vasoconstrictor substance in the serum. Experimental observations on the vasoconstrictor action of blood serum led Janeway et al. (1918) to stress the role of platelets in the development of this phenomenon. In 1948 Rapport et al., isolated the vasoconstrictor substance from beef serum and named it serotonin. In 1951, Hamlin and Fischer synthetized serotonin and confirmed it to be 5-hydroxytryptamine. Erspamer and Asero (1952) had previously extracted a substance called enteramine and indicated that it was a specific hormone of the enterochromaffin cell system. They identified the substance as 5-hydroxytryptamine and noted that it was formed in the Kulchitsky cells of the intestinal mucosa. Until the definitive study of Erspamer and Asero there had been many theories concerning the secretory activity of the Kulchitsky cells. The substance was considered to have an endocrine function by some; others considered its action to be exocrine, absorptive, or excretory. The erroneous belief that these cells had an exocrine function was based on the observation by Toro (1929) that these cells increased during starvation as well as feeding. Cordier (1926) found that applications of acid and alkali to the mucous membrane of animals, variations in diet, or the administration of intravenous pilocarpine caused a release of granules with discharge into the gut without an increase in argentaffin granules.

Other early investigators thought that these cells had an endocrine function and referred to the carcinoid tumors derived from them as endocrine tumors. Ciaccio (1906) thought that these cells produced epinephrine, while Parat (1924) considered them a source of secretin. Masson (1938) considered that these cells had a neuroendocrine function with production of a chemical substance that could activate local symphathetic nerve endings, thereby providing synaptic mediation. Eros (1932) suggested that these cells were related to the islets of Langerhans, equating their endocrine function with the theory that these cells were derived from pancreatic rests.

Jacobson (1939) considered these cells to have a hematopoietic function. He considered that the substance secreted by these cells was necessary for the prevention of pernicious anemia. He based his conclusions on the postmortem studies of twelve patients with pernicious anemia in whom he noted an absence or reduction of these cells. This work was refuted by Gillman (1942), who studied a series of Bantu within one hour of death in whom there was no evidence of pernicious anemia and yet no argentaffin cells were present in the stomach. Weisburg and Schaefer (1952) studied a large series of carcinoid tumors in the literature and rejected the view that the Kulchitsky cells were in any way similar to the glucagon-secreting alpha cells or the major secretions of the cell. The studies of Erspamer and Asero provided the turning point in the conception of the functions of the Kulchitsky cells and the endocrine nature of carcinoid tumors. Their views were strengthened when Thorson et al. (1954) described a malignant carcinoid of the small intestine with metastases to the liver. The clinical manifestations included valvular disease of the right side of the heart with pulmonary stenosis and tricuspid regurgitation without septal defects, peripheral vasomotor symptoms, bronchoconstriction, and an unusual type of cyanosis. This provided the first correlation between the clinical manifestations and the underlying pathologic findings, although the conditions had been described previously by Bjorck et al. (1952), Isler and Hedinger (1953), and Rosenbaum et al. (1953). The earliest cases with the carcinoid syndrome had, however, been described by Sir Maurice Cassidy (1931). He presented two patients before the Royal Society of Medicine with a diagnosis of metastatic carcinoma. In one of the patients pulmonary stenosis was found at subsequent autopsy, but Cassidy erroneously believed that the vascular phenomena were attributable to malignant replacement of the adrenal glands despite the fact that at postmortem the adrenal glands were demonstrably uninvolved.

In 1937, Hamperl distinguished two varieties of bronchial adenoma, the one being cylindromatous and the other carcinoid. He demonstrated that the latter could also occasionally be a cause of the carcinoid syndrome. Hamperl maintained that the carcinoid variety of bronchial adenoma, unlike appendiceal carcinoids, did not contain argentaffin cells. This assertion was proved invalid by Holley (1946), Feyrter (1959), and Williams and Azzopardi (1960). It is now accepted that the carcinoid variety of bronchial adenoma is little different from carcinoids arising elsewhere and is capable of giving rise to the carcinoid syndrome.

In 1953, Lembeck isolated 5-hydroxytryptamine from a carcinoid tumor. Pernow and Waldenstrom (1957) noted elevated levels of serotonin in the blood and urine of two patients with malignant carcinoid tumors in whom paroxysmal flushing and other symptoms were attributable to circulating 5-hydroxytryptamine and histamine. In 1955, Sjoerdsma et al. noted increased levels of urinary 5-hydroxyindoleacetic acid in the urine as reflection of the endocrine aspect of the functioning carcinoid tumors. This technique provided a simple test for the diagnosis of metastatic carcinoids. Sjoerdsma et al. (1960) used ^{14}C-tagged tryptophan to elucidate the pathway of serotonin production as well as its breakdown to 5-hydroxyindoleacetic acid. The inhibition of serotonin synthesis by alpha-methyldopa resulted in an associated increase in urinary 5-hydroxytryptophan.

Oates and Butler (1967), in an analysis of the pharmacologic and endocrine aspects of the carcinoid syndrome, demonstrated that the clinical manifestations were attributable to marked liver invasion by metastatic carcinoid tumor with the production of five pharmacologically active agents by the tumor:

1. 5-hydroxytryptamine (serotonin)
2. 5-hydroxytryptophan
3. kallikrein
4. histamine
5. Adrenocorticotrophic Hormone

Although the excessive elaboration of serotonin provided a conventional explanation for the clinical manifestations of the carcinoid syndrome, it became apparent that the intravenous injection of serotonin, though it might duplicate some of the clinical manifestations, did not precipitate episodes of flushing. The studies of Robertson et al. (1962) and consideration of the role of pressor amines and the carcinoid flush by Levine and Sjoerdsma (1963) suggested that an alternate biochemical explanation was necessary in the pathogenesis of the flushing syndrome.

Mengel (1965) reviewed the therapy of the malignant carcinoid syndrome and showed that the use of decarboxylase, hydroxylase, and serotonin inhibitors could relieve the gastrointestinal symptoms but not the flushing episodes. Schneckloth et al. (1957) showed that catecholamines could activate cutaneous flushing in carcinoid patients, while Hilton and Lewis (1956) demonstrated that catecholamines could release a kinin peptide from the perfused salivary gland. Oates et al. (1964) demonstrated the release of a kinin peptide in the carcinoid syndrome, and confirmed that hepatic kinin levels were elevated. He extracted precursors from carcinoid tumors and demonstrated that the infusion of bradykinin would induce flushing in carcinoid patients.

5-Hydroxytryptamine (Serotonin)

In his review of the biochemistry of 5-hydroxytryptamine, Dalgliesh (1956) demonstrated that tryptophan, an amino acid occurring in meat, fish, eggs, and milk products as well as cereals, is converted to 5-hydroxytryptophan (5-HTP) and the 5-HTP is converted to 5-hydroxytryptamine (5-HT) by the enzyme 5-hydroxytryptophan decarboxylase (5-HTPD). Tryptophan is normally metabolized in the liver with the production of niacin and protein. Only 1% is diverted to the production of serotonin, which is mainly found in blood platelets. Although the production of 5-HT may be somewhat dependent on the tryptophan intake, in the presence of carcinoid tumor metastases up to 60% of dietary tryptophan may be converted into serotonin. 5-hydroxytryptamine is derogated to 5-hydroxyindoleacetic acid (5-HIAA) by the enzyme monoamine oxidase (Figure 2).

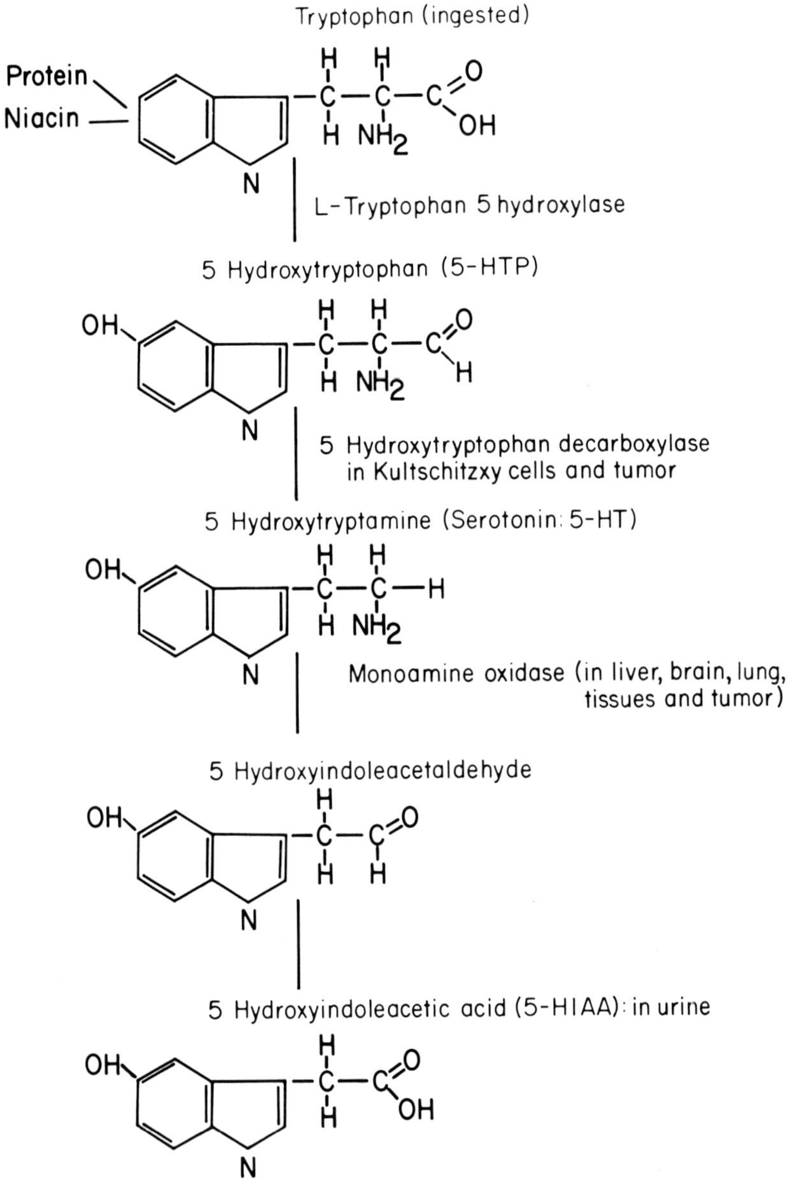

Carcinoid Tumors

Fig. 2: Metabolic pathway of serotonin.

After tryptophan has been hydroxylated to 5-HTP, the 5-HTP is absorbed by the Kulchitsky cells of the crypts of Lieberkühn in the intestine, lungs, and brain. The presence of the "universal enzyme" 5-HTPD converts 5-HTP to 5-hydroxytryptamine (serotonin). The serotonin is then released from the Kulchitsky cells into the bloodstream where it is bound by the platelets. The platelets remove the serotonin from the plasma thereby maintaining a concentration many hundreds of times higher than the surrounding tissues. The serotonin is also stored to a lesser extent in the mast cells, which also contain histamine, heparin, and hyaluronic acid. Serotonin is subsequently deaminated by monoamine oxidase in the liver as well as the lung, kidneys, and brain to 5-hydroxyacetaldehyde, which is then excreted in the urine in the form of 5-hydroxyindoleacetic acid. Gastric carcinoids may on occasion be deficient in aromatic amino acid decarboxylase and, as demonstrated by Oates and Sjoerdsma, could result in a high concentration of 5-HTP in the serum instead of 5-HT, which remains normal. An increase of urinary 5-HTP is associated with elevated urinary 5-HT as a result of the presence of kidney decarboxylase, as well as appropriate elevation of 5-HIAA.

Reserpine causes a release of 5-HT from its stores in the gastrointestinal tract, platelets, and brain, and, it is then rapidly metabolized by monoamine oxidase.

The Effects of Serotonin (5-HT)

Cardiovascular System

In a study of the effects of serotonin on arterial pressure, Page and McCubbin (1953) showed that 5-HT is amphibaric. It has a direct peripheral vasoconstrictor action leading to a pressor response. As serotonin is also a peripheral inhibitor of neurogenic vasoconstriction, a depressor response occurs if the serotonin effect is induced while the patient is in a state of excessive vasoconstriction.

Renal Effects

Serotonin causes a reduction in glomerular filtration due to a fall in renal blood flow. It further reduces urine output by enhancing tubular reabsorption of water.

Carcinoid Tumors

Hematopoietic Effects

In view of the vasoconstrictive action of serotonin on small vessels after its release from platelets, Page (1958) has implicated it as an important factor in the coagulation process. It also acts as an anti-thrombin antagonist and may act as a fibrinolytic agent in blocking the conversion of fibrinogen into fibrin.

Pulmonary Effects

Serotonin induces bronchial constriction with wheezing and dyspnea, and as a result of the pulmonary vascular vasoconstriction, this leads to the development of pulmonary hypertension. It has been suggested that in pulmonary embolism the possible release of serotonin would explain the development of pulmonary hypertension and concomitant systemic hypotension.

Gastrointestinal Effects

Serotonin increases the motility of the small intestine and the proximal colon and thereby induces diarrhea. The effect is mediated by direct smooth-muscle stimulation via receptors in the postganglionic parasympathetic neurons. This effect is not blocked by atropine or hexamethonium.

Although serotonin does not increase gastric acidity, its production has been invoked as a possible factor in the postgastrectomy dumping syndrome. The presence of increased concentration of peripheral and portal blood levels of serotonin has been associated with postgastrectomy episodes of flushing, sweating, cramps, and diarrhea. It is possible that a rapid shift of a hyperosmolar solution into the small intestine causes a release of serotonin from the Kulchitsky cells. The serotonin that is released from the gut finds its way into the portal circulation and from there to the peripheral circulation to cause its systemic effects.

Central Nervous System Effects

Serotonin is normally found in the central nervous system but does not cross the blood-brain barrier; thus, none is found in the spinal fluid of patients with elevated plasma serotonin. As Rauwolfia drugs produce depletion of serotonin in the brain, this may provide a biochemical explanation for the behavioral changes that are associated with changes in the serotonin concentration in brain tissue.

Kinins

The blood usually contains large quantities of kimogen, a kinin precursor, which under appropriate circumstances might release large amounts of kinins. The carcinoid tumors have been shown to release the enzyme kallikrein that catalyzes the release of a vasoactive kinin from its inactive precursor. Oates et al. (1964) have demonstrated that these kinins can produce hypotension, contract smooth muscle, increase blood flow, and incite pain. Kinins are derived from an alpha-2-globulin which is produced in the liver. The kinins are polypeptides consisting of many amino acids.

Bradykinin is a nonapeptide with nine amino acids arranged in a straight chain with arginine situated at the N and C terminals of the chain. Lysyl bradykinin (kallidin) has ten amino acids; the tenth is lysine. The bradykinins are inactivated by a series of enzymes known as kininases that break the nonapeptide into smaller peptides and amino acids (Figure 3).

Kallikrein (*kallikreas*, pancreas) is a hypotensive agent first derived from the pancreas but also found to occur in the salivary glands, plasma, and urine. Several different types of kallikreins have been demonstrated by paper chromatography and by trypsin inactivation.

Kinin activity may be monitored by a bioassay technique that measures its contractile effect on guinea pig ileum or its contractility effect on rat uterine muscle segments during estrus. Activity

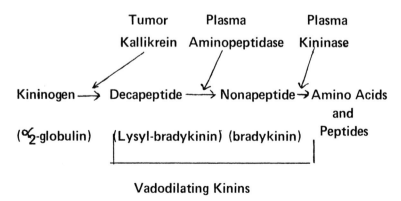

Fig. 3: Diagrammatic representation of kinin metabolism.

may also be measured by a radioimmunoassay technique in which the reaction of kinin with a bradykinin antibody is measured using a micro-complement fixation procedure.

Plasma kallikrein releases bradykinin, but the carcinoid kallikrein releases lysyl bradykinin (kallidin).

Effects of Kinins

Kinins have a vasodilatory effect in humans with diminution of peripheral vascular resistance leading to a fall in blood pressure. It is vasodilatory to the coronary and cerebral circulations and probably mediates in the cutaneous flushing occurring in patients with metastatic carcinoid tumors. Oates et al. (1964) have confirmed that injection of synthetic bradykinin produces cutaneous flushes in patients with carcinoid tumors.

Bradykinin is a powerful bronchoconstrictor. It is uncertain whether kinins play a role in intestinal motility, but significant amounts of kallikreinogen have been found in the intestinal mucosa (Eros, 1932).

The intravenous administration of bradykinin increases human renal blood flow but reduces the glomerular filtration rate and increases sodium excretion.

Chapter 3

Pathology of Carcinoids

Despite the early erroneous conclusions regarding the pathologic nature of the carcinoid tumor, Aschoff, in 1911, recognized that the carcinoid tumor could be malignant. In 1943, Dockerty and Ashburn reported 13 cases of ileal carcinoid tumors in which there were metastases. The rarity of carcinoid tumors has resulted in limitations in our knowledge and understanding of its pathological and clinical characteristics. This section attempts to provide a comprehensive picture of the pathologic, microscopic, and electron microscopic patterns of the carcinoid tumors and to relate these to their clinical patterns and natural history.

The carcinoid is generally a small tumor that arises from the argentaffin or Kulchitsky cells and may originate wherever these cells are found. The tumor may arise from any structure derived from the primitive entoderm and has been reported in teratomas of the ovary that contain entodermal elements.

In this study of 135 patients with gastrointestinal carcinoids, 35 patients (26%) had tumors 1–2 cm in diameter and 25 (11%) had tumors larger than 2 cm. It is noteworthy that there is a direct relationship between size, local invasiveness, and presence of nodal and distant metastases (Table 4).

The carcinoid tumor commences as a submucous plaque within the wall of the intestine and may be proliferative or annular in character. There is submucosal thickening around the raised nodule, which may be polypoid or sessile (Figure 4). Only rarely does superficial ulceration occur. When present, it may cause profuse gastrointestinal bleeding (Figure 5).

Carcinoid Tumors

Table 4. Extent of Disease

Location	Size	No.	Overt Malignancy No.	Overt Malignancy %	Pathologic Features Invasion	Metastases Nodes	Metastases Distant
Rectum	Less than 1 cm	25	3	12	1	2	0
	1–1.9 cm	6	3	50	2	0	2
	2 cm or larger	6	5	83	5	1	4
	Total	37	11	30	8	3	6
Jejunoileum	< 1 cm	20	6	30	6	1	0
	1–1.9 cm	12	12	100	12	8	2
	> 2 cm	5	5	100	5	5	5
	Total	37	23	62	23	14	7
Stomach	< 2 cm	5	0	0	0	0	0
	> 2 cm	5	5	100	5	5	3
	Total	10	5	50	5	5	3
Duodenum	< 2 cm	10	0	0	0	0	0
	> 2 cm	2	2	100	2	2	1
	Total	12	2	17	2	2	1
Colon	< 1 cm	1	0	0	0	0	0
	1 to 1.9 cm	2	2	100	2	1	1
	> 2 cm	7	7	100	7	7	6
	Total	10	9	90	9	8	7
Appendix	< 1 cm	29	10	34	10	0	0

NOTE: 135 carcinoid tumors of gastrointestinal tract L.S.U. affiliated hospitals.

Section of the tumor demonstrates it to be hard with a yellow coloration which may vary from pale yellow to grayish brown. The yellow color is a result of its cholesterol content and, when present, makes diagnosis of this tumor reasonably easy. Some tumors may, however, be unpigmented, but this does not affect the degree of malignancy or potential biochemical activity.

Carcinoids were found to be multiple in 40% of our patients with jejunoileal tumors and in 8% of patients with rectal lesions. Multiplicity was not a feature, however, of tumors in other locations. Each tumor is generally round and eccentrically located in the gastrointestinal tract. The frequent association of smooth-muscle hypertrophy in the vicinity of the tumor probably represents a local response to 5-HT secretion.

Although each tumor may appear to be well circumscribed and encapsulated, microscopic examination demonstrates that local infiltration and extension proceeds into the deeper layers with perineural and perilymphatic infiltration (Figure 6). Invasion of the lymphatic channels and blood vessels may occasionally be found. The pace of tumor growth is slow, and pathologic expression of malignancy tends to occur in progressive fashion with invasion of muscularis first, then gradual extension to the serosa, at which time intramural lymphatics become involved. Subsequent to the serosal involvement, extension to the surrounding structures and mesentery becomes apparent. Lymph node metastases usually develop when the tumor size exceeds 1 cm in diameter, at which time demonstrable muscular invasion is also apparent.

Among the 37 patients with rectal carcinoids in this series, there were 2 patients with carcinoids smaller than 1 cm in diameter who presented with metastases to the regional nodes in the absence of muscular invasion. There is an apparent paradox in that patients in the rectal group had a higher incidence of distant than regional nodal metastases. This is attributable to the fact that resection was not performed in several patients studied, and distant metastases were discovered at exploration without the ability to study the status of the regional nodes.

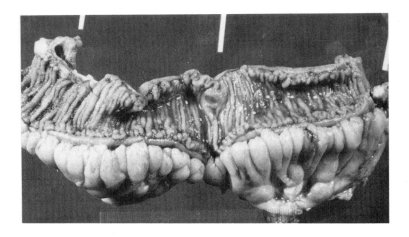

Fig. 4: Resected segment of ileum with several discrete sessile carcinoid tumors.

Carcinoid Tumors

Our study leads to the conclusion that carcinoid tumors should be considered malignant when either muscular invasion or metastases are found. Of our series of 135 cases, 50 (35%) are thus defined as representing malignant carcinoids. In the clinical group of 106 patients, 43 (41%) had carcinoids that, by these criteria, qualified for malignant status. In the autopsy group, only 7 (24%) were malignant. It becomes apparent that the larger the tumor, the more likely is its malignancy propensity.

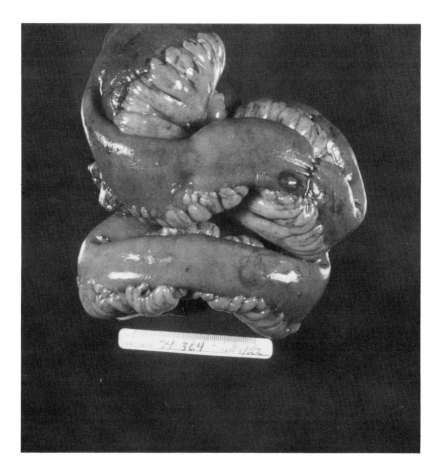

Fig. 5: Resected segment of ileum with contained blood consequent to massive bleeding from a carcinoid tumor. Note the multiple subserosal extensions.

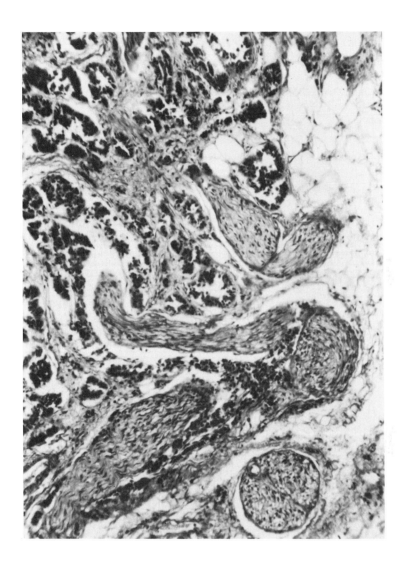

Fig. 6: Histologic pattern of carcinoid tumor with rosette arrangement and perineural invasion (H and E, x 120).

Carcinoid Tumors

Table 5. Variable Effect of Size on Malignant Propensities

Location	No.	Tumor: 1 cm +		Overt Malignancy	
		No.	%	No.	%
Colon	10	9	90	9	90
Jejunoileum	37	17	46	23	62
Stomach	10	6	60	5	50
Rectum	37	12	32	11	30
Duodenum	12	3	25	2	17

NOTE: 135 carcinoid tumors of gastrointestinal tract L.S.U. affiliated hospitals.

At each segmental level of the gastrointestinal tract, there is a correlative relationship between the tumors that were 1 cm in diameter or larger and the presence of malignant characteristics (Table 5).

Nodal metastases may be larger than the primary lesion. The most common sites for distant metastases were found to be the liver with later involvement of the lungs. Bone, skin, ovary, breast, pancreas, spleen, heart, adrenal, kidney, thyroid, pleura, testes, prostate, and cervix may all be affected by hematogenous spread.

Site Distribution

The distribution of carcinoid tumors within the respective locales in the gastrointestinal tract is demonstrated in Tables 6 and 7. It is interesting to note that the middle third of the rectum, i.e., 5 to 8 cm from the anal verge, provided the locale for 57% of the rectal carcinoids, and that 50% of this group demonstrated malignant features. Of the rectal carcinoids 43% were situated in the proximal and distal thirds of the rectum, yet malignant features were present in only 7% of this group.

A fibroblastic desmoplastic response to the tumor and its biochemical secretions leads to kinking of the bowel and the development of peritoneal adhesions, which may lead to intestinal obstruc-

Table 6. Extrarectal
Carcinoids: Site Distribution

Jejunoileum (37)	
Jejunum	5
Ileum	29
Jejunum + ileum	3
Stomach (10)	
Antrum	10
Duodenum (12)	
1st portion	10
2nd portion	2
Colon (10)	
Cecum	5
Descending colon	1
Sigmoid	4
Appendix (29)	
Base	2
Mid	4
Tip	23

NOTE: 135 carcinoid tumors of gastrointestinal tract L.S.U. affiliated hospitals.

tion. Mesenteric vascular spasm and a subadventitial fibroblastic
reaction may occur as a response to locally secreted serotonin. This
may compromise bowel vascularity with the development of local
infarction and gangrene of segments of the small intestine. Anthony
(1970) described segmental ileal necrosis in five patients as a result
of proliferation of elastic tissue in the adventitia of both the arteries
and veins.

Associated Malignant Neoplasms

It is noteworthy that although patients with colon carcinoids in this
series did not have associated malignant neoplasms, such an association occurred at every other site (Table 8).

Carcinoid Tumors

Table 7. Rectal Carcinoids:
Site Distribution

Level	No.	Malignant Features
11 cm	1	0
10 cm	5	1
9 cm	3	0
8 cm	3	2
7 cm	6	4
6 cm	7	2
5 cm	4	2
4 cm	3	0
3 cm	1	0
2 cm	2	0
Unspecified	2	0
Total	37	11

NOTE: 135 carcinoid tumors of gastrointestinal tract
L.S.U. affiliated hospitals.

A study of those cases where carcinoids and carcinoma coexisted delineates two specific patterns:

1. those in which a sharp line of demarcation exists between the two tumors
2. those in which a zone of transition can be defined

Table 8. Associated Malignant
Neoplasms

Site	No.	%
Rectum (37)	12	32
Jejunoileum (37)	14	37
Stomach (10)	2	20
Duodenum (12)	3	25
Colon (10)	0	0
Appendix (29)	4	13
Total (135)	35	26

NOTE: 135 carcinoid tumors of gastrointestinal tract L.S.U. affiliated hospitals.

It is unlikely that the carcinoid tumor represents a variant of adenocarcinoma; each of the two tumors probably has an independent origin in response to the same carcinogenic stimulus. The carcinoid develops from the Kulchitsky cells and the adenocarcinoma originates from the mucous cells of the intestinal epithelium.

This theory of separate cell origin is reinforced by the presence of argentaffin granules in the carcinoid portion of the tumor and its absence from the carcinomatous component. The sharp line of demarcation between the two tumors suggests that although their collision occurred fortuitously it may represent transition from carcinoid to adenocarcinoma.

Hernandez and Reid (1969) have questioned whether carcinoid tumors do, indeed, arise from the Kulchitsky cells and have suggested that mucosal cells may be derived from undifferentiated totipotential cells. Genetic determinants then direct the differentiation into mucous or argentaffin cells, thereby leading to the development of a mucous-secreting adenocarcinoma, a carcinoid tumor, or a composite tumor. Histochemical studies have, however, unequivocally confirmed that the argentaffin cells are derived from a neuroectodermal origin and tend to confirm the separate cell origin, each cell responding in its own way to an oncogenic stimulus.

Microscopic Patterns

Hematoxylin and eosin stains provide adequate information regarding the cytology and cellular patterns of carcinoid tumors. It is apparent that the tumor has no capsule. The cells are uniformly small in size and polypoid in shape. The cellular nuclei are round or oval and are centrally located within the eosinophilic cytoplasm that frequently contains lipid vacuoles. Although the nuclear membranes stand out prominently, each cell membrane is delicate and ill defined. Mitoses are rarely found.

Characteristic patterns of cellular arrangement are seen. The uniformly cuboidal or low columnar cells form solid nests or narrow cords of cells infiltrating between muscle layers. They stimulate a fibroblastic response that provides an interspersed fibroblastic stroma (Figure 7).

The cells may be arranged in alveolar clusters, and pseudorosette

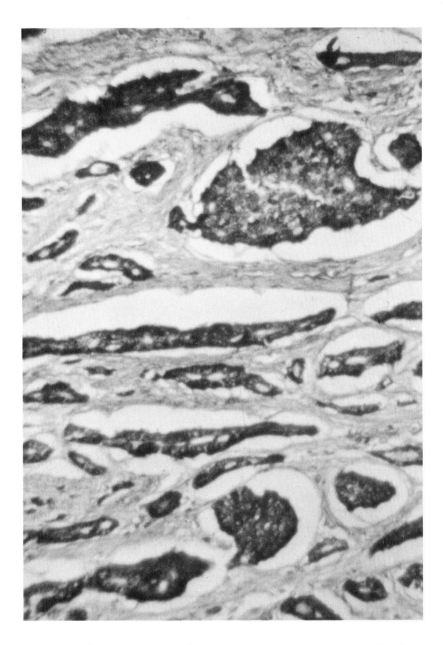

Fig. 7: Histologic appearance of carcinoid tumor demonstrating palisade arrangement of cell with desmoplastic reaction leading to deposition of collagen fibres (Masson stain, x 150).

or acinar formations are frequently seen (Figure 8). Aggressive infiltration or *degeneration* may be noted with associated *hyaline* or fatty changes, while vascular and perineural lymphatic invasion is frequently present. A trabecular pattern may be seen on occasion, the cell groups being divided by bands of dense stroma.

In addition to the stippled or punctate cytoplasmic chromatin, the acidophilic cytoplasm frequently contains basilar granules that are amenable to histochemical study.

In view of the absence of hyperchromaticity of the nuclei and the general absence of mitotic figures, the distinction between benign and malignant forms needs to be expressed in terms of invasiveness.

McDonald (1956) has suggested that carcinoid tumors be categorized as:

1. noninvasive: confined to the submucosa and mucosa
2. invading muscle of bowel wall
3. invading lymphatics or regional nodes
4. invading blood vessels with spread to distant organs

The clinical implications of these microscopic distinctions are important. In the noninvasive type or where invasion is confined to the muscle coats only, segmental bowel resection is adequate. If there is associated spread to lymph nodes, local resection must be complemented by lymph node dissection. In patients with distant metastatic spread, local resection of the primary tumor and removal of lymph nodes is highly desirable. As much bulk of metastatic tumor as possible should be removed not only to deal with the possible local complications but also to remove a source of biochemical secretion with potent clinical effects.

The frequency with which carcinoids are found to be multiple in the gastrointestinal tract (Figure 9) provides another significant challenge to the surgeon because of the need for more extensive resection than required by a single tumor. It should be borne in mind that the associated presence of an adenocarcinoma may require additional considerations regarding the strategy of surgical resection.

Histochemical Reactions of Carcinoid Tumors

The work of Lillie and Glenner (1960) has indicated that carcinoid tumors do not react identically to special stains. Those arising from

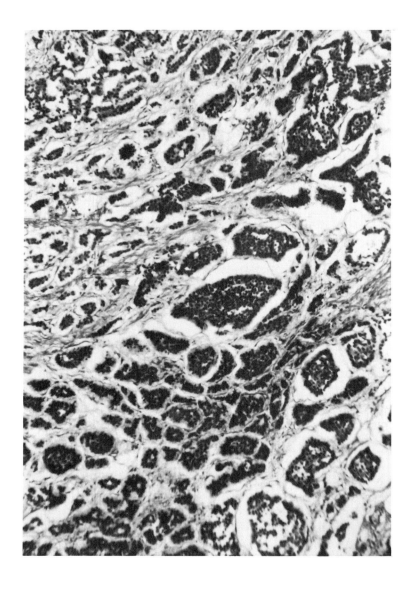

Fig. 8: Histologic pattern of carcinoid tumor with alveolar arrangement of cells (H and E, x 120).

foregut and midgut derivatives (stomach, small intestine, and right colon) usually react to silver, providing an argentaffin reaction. Some require exposure to a reducing agent before precipitating silver representing an argyrophilic reaction.

Carcinoid tumors arising from hindgut derivatives (left colon and rectum) rarely react with silver (Table 9).

The Argentaffin Reaction

This is a one-step reduction of silver salts by the cellular granules without the need for previous exposure of the tissues to reducing agents. The cells are exposed to silver solution, permitting a direct reduction, and any excess silver is removed by treating the tissues with sodium thiosulfate. The argentaffin reaction is positive only with cells arising from the enterochromaffin system and is decreased or destroyed by postmortem autolysis or by failure to provide prompt formaldehyde fixation. Reserpine therapy causes degranulation of the enterochromaffin system with depletion of serotonin.

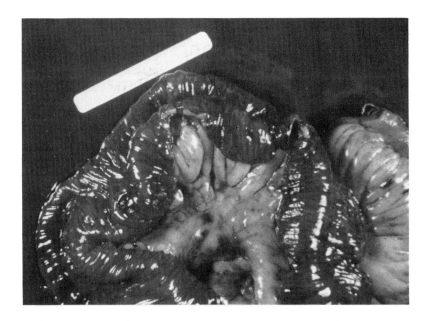

Fig. 9: Resected ileal segment with 26 distinct carcinoid tumors.

Table 9. Reactive Characteristics and Distribution

		Argyrophil	Argentaffin	Nonreaction	Total
	Bronchus	6	0	4	10
	Stomach	4	1	9	14
	Prox. duod.	1	0	4	5
FOREGUT	Pancreas	0	1	1	2
	Total	11	2	18	31
	Small int.	2	1	0	3
	Appendix and cecum	0	12	2	14
	Right colon	2	0	1	3
MIDGUT	Total	4	13	3	20
HINDGUT AND CLOACA	Left colon and rectum	0	0	11	11
	Total	15	15	32	62

NOTE: 135 carcinoid tumors of gastrointestinal tract L.S.U. affiliated hospitals.

The Argyrophilic Reaction
This is a two-step reduction of silver salts by the cellular granules. The tissue is exposed to a reducing solution so that the cytoplasmic granules are brought to a reduced state. The reduced tissue granules then act as an oxidizing agent, which, by donating an electron, is capable of reducing silver salts to the metallic silver. Any excess silver is subsequently removed by sodium thiosulfate. The argyrophilic reaction demonstrates the presence of both argyrophilic and argentaffin granules. Although this reaction is destroyed by postmortem autolysis, it is not affected by reserpine. The argyrophilic reaction is not specific and may be positive for tissue elements that are not part of the enterochromaffin system.

The Ferric-Ferricyanide Reaction
Carcinoid tumors may occasionally fail to stain with silver as an expression of biologic idiosyncrasy. In such cases, the ferric-ferricyanide reduction technique will demonstrate carcinoid gran-

ules and will be positive in tumors that are histologically carcinoid but, fail to stain with silver. This histochemical identification is rendered negative by the previous administration of reserpine.

Ninhydrin Reaction
This organic compound reacts with free amino acids, proteins, proteose, and peptones, producing a blue color; it is useful in demonstrating carcinoid granules.

Alkaline Diazo-Coupling Reaction
Lillie et al. (1961) tested 30 diazonium salts and noted that the enterochromaffin granules could be demonstrated by various diazonium salts. Although the exact mechanism is unclear, it was considered to be pH dependent and enzymatically induced. P-anisidine diazonium salts were found to be the best of the various salts tested, although, in several cases, the granules stained best with p-nitroaniline.

Indophenol Condensation
When phenol combines with dimethyl-p-phenylenediamine in the presence of an oxidizing agent, a blue green dye is produced. The argentaffin granules contribute to this phenolic group for the appropriate reaction to occur. This reaction also accounts for the carcinoid granules accepting hematoxylin and similar dyes.

Ultraviolet Light: Fluorescence and Absorption
Carcinoid granules exposed to ultraviolet light absorb certain portions of the light spectrum. The work of Eros (1932) and Jacobson (1939) has shown that the carcinoid granules have a fluorescent spectrum with two bands that peak at 6100 angstroms (610 μ) and 5550 A. Dolezel et al. (1969) attributed the fluorescence to the ability of monoamine to condense formaldehyde and thereby form carbolinic chains. Fluorescence is thus demonstrated in formalin-fixed tissues.

If an ultraviolet monochromatic light is passed through granule-containing tissues, its absorption is measurable by spectrophotometry. Carcinoid granules have a maximum absorption at 2700 A.

Electron Microscopy

Carcinoid tumor tissue was prepared for electron-microscopic examination after fixing small blocks of tissue in buffered 3% glutaraldehyde solution followed by postfixation in osmium tetroxide. The blocks were then imbedded in epon, and thin sections were stained with uranyl acetate and lead citrate and examined with a Phillip's MU 200 microscope. Portions of tissue were also fixed in 10% formalin, and the bulk tissue was treated by the Fontana method for demonstration of argentaffin granules. The bulk tissue was then postfixed in palade-sucrose, imbedded in epon, and after staining with uranyl acetate and lead citrate electron-microscopic examination was conducted.

Examination of carcinoid tissue demonstrates the cell cytoplasm to be electron translucent. The cells have pseudopod-like processes extending $1-2$ μ from the cells and insinuating themselves between adjacent exocrine cells. The cell cytoplasm has scanty endoplasmic

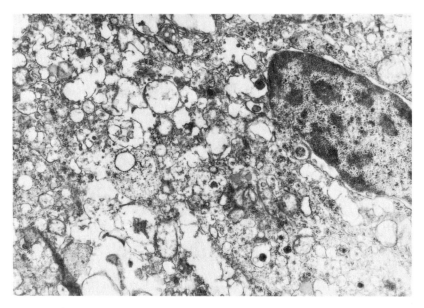

Fig. 10: Electron-microscopic study of carcinoid tumor demonstrates mitochondria and absence of endoplasmic reticulum. Note the chromatin clumps in the nucleus, attesting to proliferative activity (stained with uranyl acetate and lead citrate, x 40,000).

reticulum but large mitochondria (Figure 10). Characteristic of carcinoid tissue are the numerous electron-dense granules scattered throughout the cytoplasm. These granules are 50–80 μ and possess an internal structure similar to the neurosecretory granules of normal adrenal medullary cells and the alpha cells of the pancreatic islets. The granules consist of an electron-dense core surrounded by a clear zone separating it from the investing membrane. The granules are scattered haphazardly throughout the cell cytoplasm, many immediately below the cell membrane (Figure 11).

The tumor cells demonstrate a variable degree of electron opacity, some being opaque, others clearer, but resembling the normal Kulchitsky cells. The carcinoid cells possess pseudopod-like processes, up to 1 μ in size, interdigitating with those of neighboring cells. Occasionally desmosomes are noted at the cell interfaces, and cytoplasmic filaments are found in some of the tumor cells.

The numerous mitochondria provide a contrast to the scanty but well-developed smooth endoplasmic reticulum. Cisternae may fuse

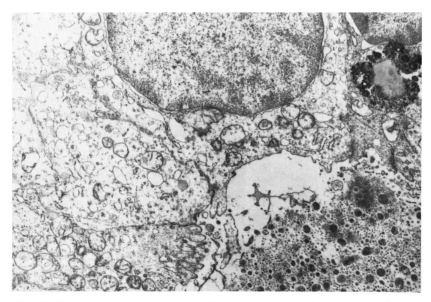

Fig. 11: Electron-microscopic study of carcinoid tumor demonstrates the discrete arrangement of the electron-dense secretory granules. Note the lipofuscin vacuole with surrounding granules (stained with uranyl acetate and lead citrate, x 34,000).

to form large, single cisternal spaces. Lysosomes are noted as aggregates of electron-dense granules bound by limiting membranes of the phagolysosomal type.

The intracellular neurosecretory granules are scattered throughout the cytoplasm, varying in diameter from 70 to 500 μ. It can be demonstrated that these granules consist of dense aggregations of fine argentaffin components (Figure 12).

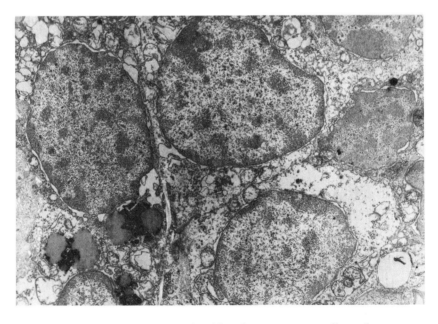

Fig. 12: Electron-microscopic study of five distinct tumor cells with intense nuclear proliferative activity. Electron-dense granules surround lipofuscin vacuoles (stained with uranyl acetate and lead citrate, x 17,000).

Chapter 4

Bronchial Carcinoids

Goldman et al. testified in 1969 to the rarity of carcinoid of the larynx in reporting the only case of such a lesion in a 73-year-old man. They described a 2-cm lesion, affecting the anterior commissure of the larynx, treated by preoperative irradiation, laryngectomy, and radical neck dissection. Mestastatic tumor was found in four nodes, and death occurred two years later from widespread metastases.

Bronchial adenomas were first recognized in 1882 when Muller described such a lesion at necropsy, and similar lesions were subsequently described by Heine (1927) and Reisner (1928). In 1930 Kramer diagnosed the condition clinically for the first time and indicated that although the lesion grew slowly malignant change might supervene.

At this time, bronchial adenomas were designated as benign glandular tumors of mucosal origin, which, by virtue of localization, rate of growth, and low level of malignancy, differed from bronchogenic carcinoma. The bronchial adenoma is a slowly growing, circumscribed neoplasm situated in the subepithelial tissues of the proximal bronchi and may be polypoid or sessile in configuration.

Histologically, the lesion is generally well differentiated. An adenoma arises from the mucous glands or ducts, and, as these are more abundant in the proximal segments of the bronchial tree, it is here that bronchial adenomata are usually located.

In 1937, Hamperl distinguished for the first time two varieties of bronchial adenoma, categorizing them as cylindroid and carcinoid.

Carcinoid Tumors

At this time, Hamperl expressed the view that the bronchial carcinoid, unlike the carcinoids of the gastrointestinal tract, did not contain argentaffin cells. The invalidity of this assertion was subsequently demonstrated by Holley (1946), Feyrter (1959), and Williams and Azzopardi (1960).

Williams and Sandler (1963) demonstrated that carcinoids could arise from any component of the primitive embryonic foregut, midgut, or hindgut. The tracheobronchial system is derivatively part of the foregut, and bronchial carcinoids resemble those in other parts of the foregut—stomach, duodenum, gall bladder—and is quite capable of giving rise to the carcinoid syndrome.

The studies of Liebow (1952) led him to categorize bronchial adenomata as carcinoids, cylindromas, and mucoepidermoid tumors.

The cylindromas, though similar to carcinoids, are paler in appearance, firmer, and on section have a moist, translucent surface. They are more likely to extend along the bronchial wall, with areas of irregular protrusion. Microscopy demonstrates that the cylindroma consists of branching acini, often lined with two layers of cells, while the acinar luminae may be traversed by cellular bridges. Large, tongue-like protrusions of cell masses may be seen, while the acini are often full of acidophil granular material that stains with mucicarmine. The cells are less uniform, smaller, and more eosinophilic than in carcinoids, and mitoses are frequently seen. The lesion is less vascular and more prone to invade cartilage, septa, and parenchyma than carcinoid tumors.

The mucoepidermoid tumor frequently secretes mucus and has a close resemblance to the mixed salivary gland tumor. This feature indicates that this tumor develops from bronchial mucous glands.

For a long time, these tumors were considered to be benign and were treated by bronchoscopic excision. Gradually the views of Goodner et al. (1961), Weiss and Ingram (1961), Zellos (1962), and Logan et al. (1970) prevailed; they stressed that local invasiveness and metastatic potential required their categorization as potentially malignant tumors. Despite a slower rate of growth and a more gradual development of metastases than bronchogenic carcinoma, a more radical operative approach is indicated.

Clinical Material

From 1948 to 1973, 28 patients with bronchial adenomas were diagnosed at Charity Hospital and Veterans Administration Hospital in New Orleans. The pathologic classification of the adenomata were: 24 (86%), the carcinoid type, 3 (11%), cylindroid, 1 (3%), a mucoepidermoid tumor.

Incidence

During this period of time, 4533 cases of primary bronchogenic tumors were seen at these state institutions, so that bronchial adenoma represented 0.6% of primary lung tumors. Naclerio and Langer (1948) indicated that bronchial adenoma accounted for 8% of all tumors of the lower respiratory tract. Sanders and Kingsley (1948) noted the incidence to be 6.9%, but Price-Thomas (1954) found the incidence to be 2%. Burcharth and Axelson (1972) described 26 patients with bronchial adenomas and noted its incidence to be 1.2% of all primary tumors. The apparent gradual reduction in the incidence of bronchial adenoma seems to be a result of the increasing incidence of bronchogenic carcinomas rather than a result of an overall reduction in the actual incidence of bronchial adenomas.

Age and Sex Incidence

In 1941, Foster-Carter, in a study of 70 cases, indicated that the highest incidence of bronchial adenoma occurred in the 31- to 40-year age group and noted that 62% occurred in females. Moersch and McDonald (1950) noted that the average age of females was 38 years, while in males it was 42 years of age. Their youngest patient was 15 years old. Zellos (1962), in a study of 40 cases of bronchial adenoma, found that half the patients were over 50 years of age. He described a 16-year-old patient whose symptoms had lasted 8 years before the diagnosis was established.

In the present series, the age and sex incidence indicated a ratio of 15 females to 13 males, representing a slight female preponderance. The average age of the female group was 45 years; the male, 54 years (Table 10).

Table 10. Bronchial Adenomas

Age	Female	Male
10–19	1	0
20–29	2	0
30–39	4	2
40–49	4	4
50–59	2	2
60–69	1	3
Over 70	1	2
Total	15	13

Clinical features resulted from the effects of bronchial obstruction, which caused distal infection, bronchiectasis, or development of a lung abscess. Recurrent episodes of pneumonia occurred in several patients.

Hemoptysis occurred in only 18% of the series. Interestingly, eight patients (29%) were asymptomatic and the condition was noted on routine chest X rays. Cough was a dominant feature in five patients, hemoptysis occurred in five, and recurrent pneumonia was the presenting feature in three patients. Weakness, chest pain, fever, and weight loss were noted in several patients. The duration of symptoms varied from six months to eight years.

A retrospective analysis of radiologic features (Figure 13) indicated the presence of a well-defined tumor in 13 patients, poorly defined areas of infiltration in 9, atelectasis as the dominant radiologic feature in 7, and lung abscess in 1 patient.

Tomography, helpful in patients with ill-defined opacities, confirmed the solid nature of the lesions. Bronchoscopic biopsy provided a positive diagnosis in 26 patients.

Cytologic examination had no diagnostic value in this series of patients; negative findings were reported in all sputum examinations, except for the presence of atypical cells in one patient. In six patients bronchial-washing examinations were performed, providing a totally negative yield. Scalene node biopsy was carried out in two patients without providing diagnostic information. An axillary node biopsy in one patient with a malignant carcinoid tumor provided evidence of the metastatic nature of the lesion.

Distribution of Bronchial Adenomas
Nineteen tumors occurred in the right bronchopulmonary tree and
nine in the left. The lobar distribution is given in Table 11.

Operative Procedures
Pneumonectomy was performed in nine cases, and lobectomy in
eight. Bronchoscopic biopsy alone was performed in seven patients,
and in four cases the tumors were examined at autopsy. Although
bronchoplastic operations or sleeve resections were not performed
in this series of patients, these more desirable procedures have been
performed in a more recent series of patients.

Associated Disease
One patient with a bronchial cylindroid adenoma had undergone
successful mastectomy for carcinoma of the breast eight years ear-

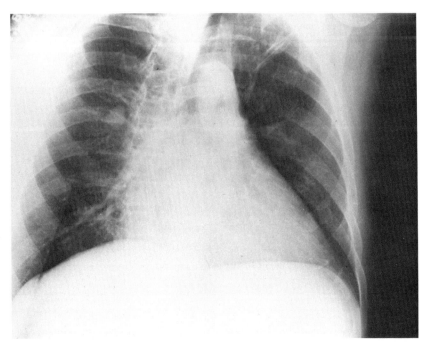

*Fig. 13: Chest X ray demonstrates discrete nodule in right parahilar region,
confirmed at bronchoscopic biopsy to be a carcinoid tumor. It was subsequently treated by right upper lobectomy.*

Table 11. Distribution of Bronchial Adenomas

	Right	Left
Upper Lobe	8	6
Middle Lobe or Lingula	4	1
Lower Lobe	5	2
Main Stem Bronchus	2	0
Total	19	9

lier. One patient with a bronchial carcinoid had histologic evidence of prostatic carcinoma after prostectomy for bladder neck obstruction. One patient had active fibrocaseous tuberculosis concurrently with the development of a bronchial carcinoid. Two patients with bronchial carcinoids had clinical evidence of endocrine abnormalities.

Incidence of Metastases
In the 17 patients who underwent resection, positive lymph node extension was found in 3. This finding did not materially affect survival. One patient with lymph node extension from a bronchial carcinoid who underwent right pneumonectomy died in the immediate postoperative period. Lymph node metastasis was found in the patient with associated advanced fibrocaseous tuberculosis with a malignant bronchial carcinoid, the condition being confirmed at autopsy. The third was in a patient who died from the effects of widespread metastases, as well as mediastinal lymph node involvement eight years after onset of the disease. In all the other resected specimens, lymph nodes were negative at pathologic examination.

The patterns of hematogenous spread indicate a predilection for the liver, adrenals, glands, bones, brains, as well as mediastinal and bronchopulmonary lymph nodes, and in one case, spread to the ipsilateral axillary nodes.

Survival
If one excludes the one operative death and the autopsy cases, there is a residual clinical group of 19 patients. One patient survived for longer than 20 years after a previous pneumonectomy for bronchial carcinoid. Nine patients survived 10 to 20 years, and in this group 4

Table 12. Bronchial Carcinoids:
Survival

Years	Number	Percent
< 1	1	5.2
1–5	2	10.4
5–9	3	16
10	3	16
10–20	9	47.2
> 20	1	5.2
Total	19	100.0

patients underwent pneumonectomy, 4 patients were treated by lobectomy, and 1 patient had refused surgery. This last case exemplifies the slow growth and low order of malignancy of the lesion.

Three patients survived 10 years. Two patients were treated by pneumonectomy, and one patient had a lobectomy. Three patients survived between 5 and 10 years; two of this group had undergone lobectomy, and one survived 7 years after refusing surgical exploration. Two patients survived between 1 to 5 years; one of these patients had a lobectomy, and the other refused surgery. One patient, after previous pneumonectomy, survived less than 1 year (Table 12).

Not only may symptoms extend over many years before the condition is diagnosed, but in the three patients who refused surgery, the radiologic existence of the lesion has been known for up to 15 years without notable progression.

Cause of Death
Analysis of the eight patients who died indicates that one postoperative death occurred after pneumonectomy in 1951. One patient survived 16 months after right lower lobectomy, death being due to a myocardial infarction. One patient died 8 years after the diagnosis of malignant carcinoid had been confirmed and surgery deemed inappropriate. Death was attributable to cerebral hemorrhage after craniotomy for a cerebral metastasis.

One patient died 24 years after surgical cure for the condition, death being due to coronary artery disease. One patient died from arteriosclerotic heart disease, and the bronchial carcinoid was an incidental autopsy finding. One patient died of advanced fibrocaseous tuberculosis, and a concomitant bronchial carcinoid was confirmed at autopsy. Death occurred in one patient 9 months after pneumonectomy for bronchial carcinoid as a result of a myocardial infarction, and one patient died 19 years after lobectomy for bronchial carcinoid as the result of an automobile accident.

Pathogenesis

In 1928, Reisner and subsequently Kramer (1930) suggested that bronchial adenomas arose from the ductal epithelium of bronchial glands. Churchill (1937) and Womack and Graham (1938) considered the origin to be from residual embryonic pulmonary tissue consisting of entodermal and mesodermal elements. They explained the resemblance of the mucoepidermoid variety of bronchial adenoma to mixed salivary gland tumors on this basis. At this time, they suggested that bronchial adenomas be considered malignant tumors.

Willis (1940) postulated the probability that these tumors arose from the mucous and mixed glands of the bronchial mucosa. Felton et al. (1953) held the view that the central and peripheral varieties of bronchial adenomas had different origins. Although they concurred that proximal lesions arose from mucous glands, they believed that the periperhal tumors arose from the lining of the epithelium. The controversy that had been extant regarding the origin and natural history of bronchial adenomas needs to be viewed in the light that clear distinction must be made between the carcinoid type, the cylindromatous variety, and the mucoepidermoid tumor. The cylindroma, also known as an adenoid cystic carcinoma, is the most malignant of the three types, arising from the basal or surface epithelium of the bronchial ducts. The term bronchial adenoma, therefore, refers to three and possibly more distinct neoplasms that differ in structure as well as in their natural history.

Pathologic Effects

Although most bronchial carcinoids fail to show argentaffin granules under light microscopy, most are argyrophilic. Williams and Sandler (1963) distinguished three carcinoid groups, based on differing embryologic derivations associated with varying biochemical characteristics distinctive for each group.

1. foregut origin: bronchus, stomach, duodenum, biliary tract, and pancreas
2. midgut origin: arising from the midduodenum to mid-transverse colon
3. hindgut origin: descending colon and rectum

The bronchial carcinoid is a smooth, globular tumor that protrudes into a proximal bronchus with its partial or complete occlusion (Figure 14). Nineteen bronchial adenomas were found on the right side, and nine tumors in the left bronchial tree. This preponderance of right-sided tumors was also represented in the carcinoid group. The bronchial obstruction may lead to the development of distal bronchiectasis (Figure 15) or recurrent pneumonia with the subsequent development of a lung abscess (Figure 16). Dyspnea with localized wheezing, emphysema, and associated bronchospasm may occur.

Although hemoptysis may be the only presenting clinical feature of the endobronchial mass, bronchoscopic examination generally discloses an intact mucous membrane without ulceration. Although the lesion is endobronchial, it generally extends beyond the bronchus, and the extrabronchial component may be large, even if the endobronchial component is quite small. The cut surface of the neoplasm may vary from a pale-pink soft tumor to a tan-colored lobulated firm lesion with its parenchymal surface covered by a connective tissue capsule (Figure 17).

In the more invasive or frankly malignant bronchial carcinoid, the capsule is poorly defined. It is noteworthy that a desmoplastic fibrous reaction or tissue necrosis is unusual, in contrast to the frequency of these features in carcinoids of the gastrointestinal tract.

Although most bronchial carcinoids have a benign clinical course with prolonged survival, even in the absence of extirpative surgery, the tumor does on occasion transgress its normal restrictive barriers with local invasiveness, infiltration of lymph nodes, and hematogenous spread. In the present series, positive lymph nodes were found in three resected specimens and in one case, spread had occurred to the axillary nodes, as well as manifesting signs of associated hematogenous spread.

When hematogenous spread does occur, the sites of predilection are liver, adrenals, brain, and bones. Although bone metastases are

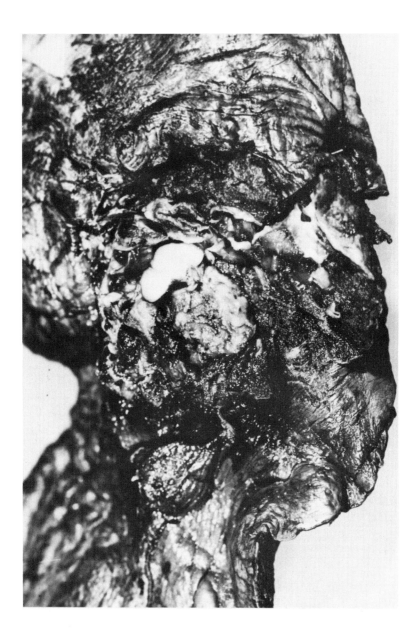

Fig. 14: Examination of the specimen after lobectomy demonstrates the endobronchial and parenchymal components of the bronchial carcinoid tumor.

rare, when they do occur, they are generally osteoblastic in nature. Pollard et al. (1962) reported an unusual case of metastasizing bronchial adenoma associated with the carcinoid syndrome and noted the presence of numerous osteoblastic lesions. Toomey and Felson (1960) noted the similarity of the osteoblastic patterns of metastatic carcinoid lesions resulting from primary tumors in both the gastrointestinal tract and the bronchial tree. In a review of 17 cases of bone metastases from carcinoid tumors, Thomas noted that the lesions were blastic in 14 cases, mixed blastic and lytic in 2, and purely lytic in only 1 case.

In one patient in our series, craniotomy with partial removal of a posterior fossa tumor confirmed the lesion to be metastatic from a malignant bronchial carcinoid. At autopsy two days later, the nature of the primary lesion was confirmed. At this time, associated sites of metastases were noted in adrenals, bones, pleura, and lymph nodes of the thorax and axilla. The duration of survival from diagnosis of the bronchial lesion had been eight years, and its failure to respond to radiotherapy over a two-year period was noteworthy.

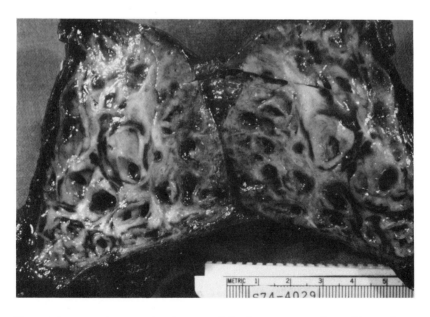

Fig. 15: Section of resected right upper lobe demonstrates bronchiectasic changes distal to an obstructive bronchial carcinoid tumor.

Carcinoid Tumors

The infrequency of associated concomitant or synchronous malignant disease in bronchial carcinoid may be contrasted with the frequent coexistence of evident carcinoma in patients with carcinoids of the gastrointestinal tract. In the present series, one patient presented with a bronchial adenoma (of the cylindroid type) 12 years

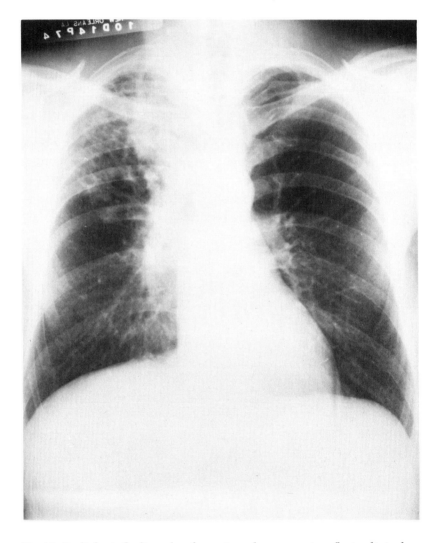

Fig. 16: Radiologic finding of atelectasis and pneumonia reflects clinical status. Bronchoscopy demonstrated a bronchial carcinoid.

after radical mastectomy for carcinoma of the breast. In the second patient prostatectomy for bladder-neck obstruction disclosed histologic evidence of prostatic carcinoma.

The presence of advanced fibrocaseous pulmonary tuberculosis in association with a malignant bronchial carcinoid in one patient in this series is worthy of note. This 56-year-old white male had been treated for pulmonary tuberculosis in 1948, and two years later routine chest X ray demonstrated that a rounded mass had developed in the left hilar region. Acid- and alcohol-fast bacilli were present in the sputum, and bronchoscopy demonstrated a lesion of the left upper lobe of the bronchus. Biopsy disclosed it to be a malignant bronchial adenoma of the carcinoid type. At autopsy two months later, the pathologic findings included advanced fibrocaseous tuberculosis and a malignant carcinoid tumor of the left upper lobe of the bronchus with metastases to the tracheobronchial, thoracic, and abdominal lymph nodes, as well as spread to the right and left lungs and pleura. Metastases were also present in the liver and both adrenal glands.

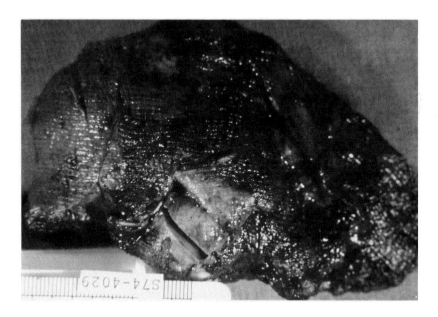

Fig. 17: Obstructive bronchial carcinoid tumor which led to atelectatic and bronchiectasic changes.

Carcinoid Tumors

Cytology

Bronchoscopic biopsy of the endobronchial lesion provides microscopic evidence of the carcinoid nature of the lesion. Sputum cytology was carried out in 13 patients and was totally negative in 12. In one patient, the presence of atypical cells was noted. Bronchial washings were studied in 6 patients, providing an entirely negative yield. Scalene node biopsy in 1 patient indicated nonspecific reticular hyperplasia. Biopsy of an axillary node demonstrated the presence of metastatic spread from a malignant bronchial carcinoid. This patient ultimately died eight years after discovery of the bronchial lesion from the effects of a cerebral metastasis.

The presence of atypical squamous cells in the sputum of one patient reflects the occasional squamous metaplasia of the surface bronchial epithelium. The absence of carcinoid cells in the sputum or in bronchial washings is attributable to the presence of a thickened reticular basement membrane and dense connective tissue that separates the surface epithelium from the underlying tumor tissue.

The Carcinoid Cell

Bensch et al. (1965) first demonstrated Kulchitsky-type cells in normal bronchi. Their ultrastructural electron-microscopic study demonstrated cells in normal human bronchial mucosa that resembled the intestinal argentaffin cells. Gmelich et al. (1967) demonstrated that these cells were incorporated between exocrine cells situated within the limiting basement membrane and could be identified by their small, dark cytoplasmic granules. Similar cells were also found between the columnar cells lining the peripheral bronchioles. It is these Kulchitsky-type cells that probably provide origin for the peripheral carcinoid tumor. The cells are particularly prominent in the larger bronchi, especially at sites of bronchial bifurcation. The argentaffin cell was originally thought to be derived from entoderm but is now generally accepted to have a neuroectodermal origin. These cells are probably derived from the neural crest and migrate to the components of the foregut, represented by bronchus, stomach, biliary tract, pancreas, and proximal half of the duodenum; the midgut, represented by the intestine, from the midduodenum to the midtransverse colon; and the hindgut, represented by descending colon and rectum. This migration commences in the 12-week fetus, occurring long before these cells mature to develop this silver reaction. The failure of some of these cells to develop the silver reaction may represent an expression of biologic idiosyncracy.

Light Microscopy

The carcinoid cell is typically uniform and small with acidophilic cytoplasm demonstrable with hematoxylin and eosin stains. Although it is quite unusual to find nuclear mitoses or argentaffin granules, the nuclei contain finely stippled chromatin.

The cells are arranged in sheets, strands, or rounded masses resembling acini. The cell groups are situated in sinusoidal vascular spaces, which may be so prominent as to suggest a hemangioma. This vascularity may lead to severe hemorrhage at bronchoscopic attempts to remove the endobronchial component of the carcinoid.

Local invasiveness may be expressed by cellular permeation of the capsule or by perivascular and perineural extension (Figure 18). Despite this connotation of malignant potential, these cases are nevertheless associated with prolonged survival. The presence of tumor cells within bronchial or paratracheal lymph nodes is not necessarily indicative of subsequent spread. Fragments of bone are occasionally noted as a result of metaplasia in portions of the isolated bronchial cartilages.

Occasionally bulky cells are seen with granular or striated cytoplasm with small nuclei which contain a network of coarse chromatin. These oncocytic cells may be interspersed with carcinoid or transitional cells.

Histologic criteria cannot be used to differentiate between benign and malignant tumors. A basis for diagnosis of malignancy must rest on the degree of local invasiveness, lymph node involvement, and metastases.

Electron Microscopy

Carcinoid tumor cells demonstrate a variable degree of electron density, with some cells demonstrating greater opacity than others. The resemblance of the tumor cells to normal Kulchitsky cells is quite striking. The carcinoid cells possess villous processes up to 1 μ in size that interdigitate with those of adjacent cells. Although mitochondria are numerous, the smooth endoplasmic reticulum is scanty, though well developed (Figure 19). Large cisternal spaces

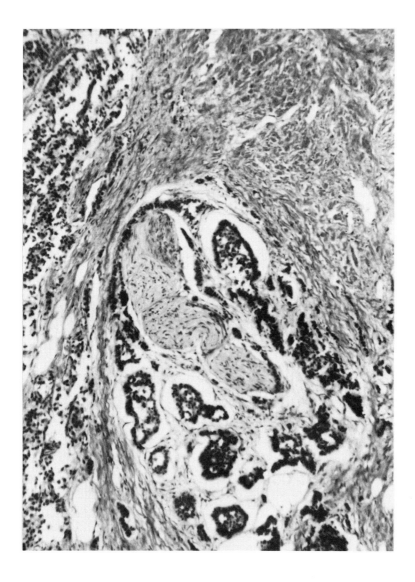

Fig. 18: Histologic appearance of bronchial carcinoid tumor with perineural and lymphatic invasion (H and E, x 150).

may be seen as a result of fusion of several smaller cisternae. Aggregations of electron-dense bodies may be seen, bound by limiting membranes of the phagolysosomal type. The lysosomal character of these cells is confirmed by their high acid phosphatase content.

Characteristic of the carcinoid cell is the presence of intracellular neurosecretory granules, 100 to 500 μ in diameter, scattered throughout the cytoplasm (Figure 20). Many granules are found directly beneath the cell membrane, and aggregations of the granules are often found in the vicinity of the Golgi apparatus. The granules are generally more numerous and are more variable in size than in Kulchitsky cells.

The electron-microscopic examination of bronchial carcinoids prepared by the Fontana silver impregnation technique of bulk-fixed tissue demonstrates that the neurosecretory granules consist of dense aggregations of fine argentaffin granules. This is in contrast to the fact that under light microscopy most bronchial carcinoids do

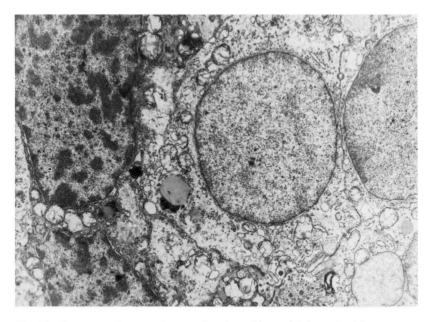

Fig. 19: Electron-microscopic examination of bronchial carcinoid tumor demonstrates variable nuclear proliferative activity. Note occasional desmosomes at cell interface. Scanty electron-dense granules present (stained with uranyl acetate and lead citrate, x 24,000).

not contain demonstrable argentaffin granules, the majority of these cells being argyrophilic. This apparent anomaly may depend on the ability of the neurosecretory granules to store its secretion with variable ability to reduce silver compounds.

Bronchial Carcinoids and Oat Cell Carcinoma

A relationship between bronchial carcinoids and oat cell bronchogenic carcinoma is suggested by the fact that the oat cell or undifferentiated carcinoma is a specific and separate entity from other bronchogenic carcinomas. It is composed of uniformly small cells with hyperchromatic nuclei and scanty stroma formation. Its cells arise from the deeper layers of the bronchial epithelium and bear a close resemblance to the normal basal cells from which the bronchial epithelium is normally regenerated. Bronchial carcinoids are

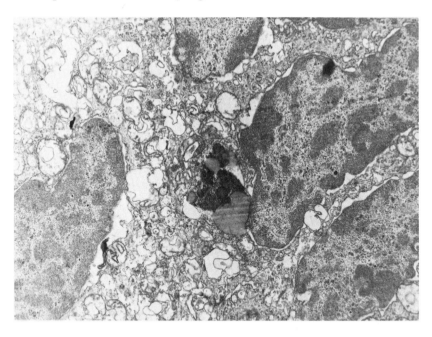

Fig. 20: Electron-microscopic study of bronchial carcinoid with intense nuclear activity. Mitochondria are numerous, but endoplasmic reticulum are absent. Electron-dense granules are clumped around a lipofuscin vacuole (stained with uranyl acetate and lead citrate, x 34,000).

usually argyrophilic but may, on occasion, be argentaffinic. Argentaffin cells are also frequently found in oat cell carcinoma.

Oat cell carcinomas frequently demonstrate the ability to exert hormonal effects. It can cause Cushing's syndrome as well as the carcinoid syndrome with urinary excretion of excessive amounts of 5-HIAA or 5-HTP. It may secrete other polypeptide hormones, justifying its inclusion as a malignant member of the apud family.

These characteristics strongly suggest that the oat cell carcinoma as well as the bronchial carcinoid originate in the Kulchitsky cells of the bronchial epithelium. They demonstrate varying patterns of malignant transformation. Bronchial carcinoids represent a locally spreading neoplasm; oat cell carcinoma, the anaplastic malignant variant.

Electron-microscopic study of oat cell tumors demonstrates neurosecretory-type granules similar to those of the carcinoid tumor, further attesting to their common origin.

Hormonal Considerations

In 1906, Ciaccio suggested that carcinoids might be biochemically active and believed erroneously that they might release epinephrine. Toenniessen (1910) emphasized the resemblance of carcinoid cell nests to the islets of Langerhans and suggested that the tumor might provide endocrine secretions.

The attempt to purify a vasoconstrictor substance from beef serum led Rapport et al. (1948) to the first isolation of serotonin. Hamlin and Fischer (1951) successfully synthesized 5-hydroxytryptamine, and in the following year Erspamer and Asero (1952) identified a substance that they named enteramine as 5-hydroxytryptamine (serotonin). They also identified the substance as the specific hormone of the enterochromaffin cell system and noted that serotonin was present in the Kulchitsky cells of the intestinal mucosa.

Lembeck (1953) first extracted serotonin from a carcinoid tumor. Within the next two years the concept of the carcinoid syndrome was recognized, as cases were described with systemic symptomatology attributable to release of excessive amounts of serotonin by intestinal carcinoid tumors with liver metastases.

Sjoerdsma et al. (1955) devised a simple screening test for the diagnosis of metastatic carcinoids when they noted an increased excretion of urinary 5-hydroxyindoleacetic acid as an expression of the hormonal function of carcinoid tumors. Sjoerdsma et al. (1960) used ^{14}C-tagged tryptophan to elucidate the pathway of serotonin production and its breakdown to 5-hydroxyindoleacetic acid. Oates and Butler (1967) in an analysis of the pharmacologic and endocrine aspects of the carcinoid syndrome demonstrated that the clinical manifestations were attributable to marked liver invasion by metastatic carcinoid tumors with the production of four pharmacologically active agents by the tumor: 5-hydroxytryptamine (serotonin), bradykinin, histamine, and ACTH. By this time, there were 159 published cases of the carcinoid syndrome. The primary tumor occurred in the small intestine in 115 of these cases.

The ability of bronchial carcinoids to cause the carcinoid syndrome was clearly demonstrated by Schneckloth et al. (1959). They described a 45-year-old male patient who underwent right lower lobectomy for a bronchial carcinoid and three months later developed facial flushing precipitated by eating. This was associated with markedly elevated urinary excretion of 5-hydroxyindoleacetic acid. Two years after lobectomy, laparotomy was performed. The liver was studded with metastatic carcinoid tissue, and three large tumor deposits were removed. Microscopy revealed morphologic characteristics similar to those noted in the previously removed pulmonary tumor.

Although flushing episodes were subsequently less frequent and less intensive, the daily range of urinary 5-HIAA remained unchanged. Autopsy after death a month later revealed massive peritonitis due to a perforated duodenal ulcer. It was noted that the right lobe was completely replaced by carcinoid tumor material that had undergone necrosis and hemorrhage, but no argentaffin granules could be found in the tumor.

The excessive production of serotonin and elevated urinary excretion of 5-HIAA is not, however, associated with the flushing component of the carcinoid syndrome. Oates et al. (1964) have demonstrated that the release of kinin peptide occurs in the carcinoid syndrome, thus probably explaining the mechanism of flushing because infusion of bradykinin can precipitate flushing in carcinoid patients. Hepatic kinin level is demonstrably elevated during flushing, and kallikrein, an enzyme which activates bradykinin from its precursor, has been isolated from carcinoid tumors.

Warner et al. (1961) reported two patients with bronchial carcinoids, in both of whom serum serotonin and urinary 5-HIAA were markedly elevated without manifestations of flushing. In both patients, one a 35-year-old male and the other a 44-year-old female, serum serotonin and urinary 5-HIAA levels were restored to normal after appropriate lobectomy. The release of serotonin by bronchial carcinoids may lead to fibrous thickening of the mitral valve, with fusion of the chordae tendineae resulting in histologic changes consistent with carcinoid valvular disease. Von Bernheimer et al. (1960) reported a case of bronchial carcinoid without metastases in which there was diffuse fibrosis of the endocardium and the valves of the left heart.

Polyendocrine Factors

Multiple adenomata of the endocrine organs was first described in a dog by Perlman (1944). Underdahl et al. (1953) first described a clinical entity that they termed pluriglandular adenomatosis. The disorder consisted of adenomatous enlargement of several endocrine glands, the usual combination affecting the pituitary, parathyroid, pancreatic islets, and adrenal glands. The familial nature of the condition was emphasized by Wermer in 1954. Marshall and Sloper (1954) described the polyendocrine syndrome in association with tumors of mesodermal origin such as a giant lipoma.

Zollinger and Ellison (1955) demonstrated the association between intractable peptic ulceration and pancreatic non-beta-cell adenomas. Several years later, Ellison (1958) indicated that 25% of a series of 72 patients with ulcerogenic tumors of the pancreas had associated adenomatosis of other endocrine organs.

In 1956, McDonald demonstrated the association of peptic ulceration with metastatic carcinoid tumors. Weichert et al. (1967) delineated the histologic similarity between carcinoid tumors and islet cell tumors and published the details of 13 patients with duodenal carcinoids and associated peptic ulceration.

Carcinoid tumors of the intestine are rarely associated with endocrine disturbances apart from the carcinoid syndrome. Fischer and Hicks (1960) and Gerber and Shields (1960) each described a patient with duodenal carcinoid tumors associated with the pluriglandular syndrome. Buse et al. (1961) described an acromegalic patient with a rectal carcinoid. No association, however, has been identified between carcinoid tumors of the lower ileum and endocrine adenomatosis.

In 1949, Goldman published a case report of a patient with a bronchial carcinoid in association with multiple pituitary and adrenal adenomata. Underdahl et al. (1953) described the association of bronchial carcinoids with multiple parathyroid adenomata and hypoglycemia. Subsequent case reports by Altman and Schutz (1959), Southern (1960), Cohen et al. (1960), Weiss and Ingram (1961), and Christy (1961) emphasized the frequent association between bronchial carcinoids, on the one hand, and acromegaly or Cushing's syndrome, on the other. Greenbaum (1960) described several members of a family with multiple parathyroid adenomata in association with bronchial carcinoids. Escovitz and Reingold (1961) described a patient with bronchial carcinoid in association with adenomas of the pituitary, parathyroid, adrenals, and pancreatic islet cells. Williams and Celestin (1962) described a patient with a carcinoid of the left lower lobe, who died from peritonitis resulting from breakdown of a gastrojejunal anastomosis subsequent to a 14-year history of peptic ulcer. Renal calculus disease was also present. In our series of 28 bronchial adenomas, 24 were of the carcinoid variety. Within this latter group, there were 2 patients with polyendocrine manifestations.

The first was a 35-year-old white male who presented with recurrent episodes of right upper lobe pneumonia. Radiologic examination of the chest demonstrated an atelectatic right upper lobe (Figure 21). Bronchoscopy visualized a polypoid lesion projecting from the upper lobe bronchus. Biopsy confirmed that it was a bronchial carcinoid. In August 1960 a successful right upper lobectomy was performed. The patient was readmitted in July 1967 with features of Cushing's disease, attributable to bilateral adrenocortical hyperplasia, associated with elevated serum 11-hydroxycorticoids. Bilateral adrenalectomy was performed in July 1967, and the patient was discharged two weeks later. At this time, serum 5-HT and urinary 5-HIAA were within normal limits. There has been no evidence of recurrence of the bronchial carcinoid on radiologic or bronchoscopic examination.

The second patient was a 34-year-old black male who was admitted in July 1943 with clinical features suggestive of a duodenal ulcer. Radiologic examination confirmed that the ulcer was in the first part of the duodenum, and gastric analysis demonstrated hyper-chlorhydria. Medical management was provided until 1946 when perforation of the ulcer led to surgical plication of the perforation. In November 1947 subtotal gastrectomy with a Billroth II reconstitu-tion and segmental resection of ileum for a small intestinal tumor was performed. Pathologic examination of the resected specimen re-vealed a healed duodenal ulcer with a duodenal carcinoid tumor. The small intestinal lesion was diagnosed as a schwannoma. Post-operative gastric analysis demonstrated normal free- and total-acid levels.

Later that year the patient redeveloped epigastric pain, and bar-ium study revealed a marginal ulcer that was confirmed at gastro-scopic examination. Vagotomy and a revision gastrectomy with an antecolic, isoperistaltic gastrojejunostomy was performed. Exami-nation of the resected specimen demonstrated a chronic jejunal

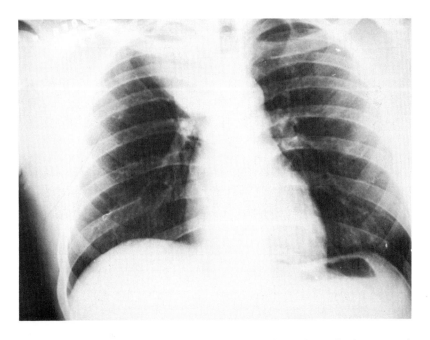

Fig. 21: Chest X ray with upper lobe atelectasis due to bronchial carcinoid.

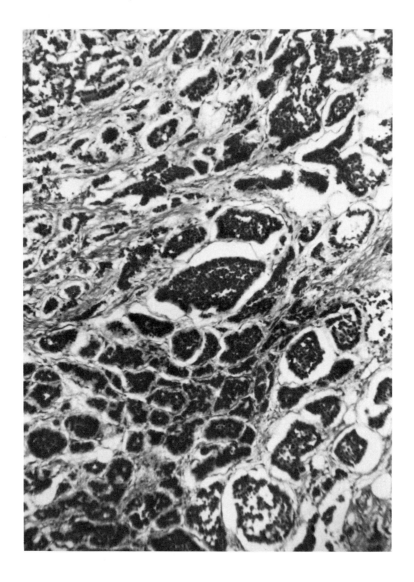

Fig. 22: Histologic examination of bronchial carcinoid demonstrates alveolar and rosette arrangement of cells (H and E, x 150).

ulcer. Recurrence of symptoms was recorded in June 1961, and recurrence of an ulcer was confirmed. A transthoracic vagotomy and a revision gastrectomy was carried out. In August 1964 recurrence of epigastric pain culminated in severe gastric bleeding requiring 26 units of blood replacement. At abdominal exploration, a marginal ulcer was found, eroding into the left lobe of the liver and into the pancreas. A gastrocolic fistula was also present. The colonic opening was repaired and a more extensive gastric resection and a gastroduodenal reconstruction was completed. Pathologic examination of the resected stomach disclosed the presence of a gastric carcinoid.

In May 1957 radiologic examination of the chest disclosed an asymptomatic 2-mm nodule in the right upper lobe, which subsequently rapidly enlarged. Bronchial washings were negative, and in July 1957 a right upper lobectomy was performed. A 2-by-0.6-cm lesion was found to arise from the wall of the right upper lobe bronchus. Histologic examination confirmed it to be a bronchial adenoma of the carcinoid type (Figure 22).

Over the ensuing 14 years the patient has had recurrent episodes of upper gastrointestinal bleeding, associated with markedly elevated urinary 5-HIAA levels. In October 1965 exploratory laparotomy yielded a lymph node that provided histologic evidence of a carcinoid metastasis. At this time, nitrogen mustard therapy was administered without notable effect. In September 1973, 16 years after the original diagnosis of carcinoid disease, gastroscopy demonstrated the presence of multiple polypoid lesions in the gastric pouch. At this time the serum gastrin level was 4702 pg/ml (normal, 0–300 pg/ml). It is of interest that the patient's brother died from the effects of a bleeding ulcer in 1971; his sister is alive but suffers from chronic peptic ulcer disease.

The association of gastric, duodenal, and bronchial carcinoids and their association with fulminating peptic ulcer disease lend emphasis to the intricate relationship between bronchial carcinoids and other endocrine conditions. There appears to be a spectrum of conditions ranging from pluriglandular adenomatosis and ulcerogenic gastrin-producing tumors that may be associated with bronchial carcinoids. The elevated levels of urinary 5-HIAA and serum gastrin in association with the bronchial carcinoid is probably attributable to the malignant tumor of the duodenum, which appears to represent another example of a carcinoid-islet cell tumor.

Chapter 5

The Gastrointestinal Tract

The Esophagus

Although argentaffin cell tumors may arise in all segments of the gastrointestinal tract, only one patient with carcinoid of the esophagus has been described in the world literature. In 1969, Brenner et al. described a diabetic 56-year-old male, previously treated for pernicious anemia, who presented with a seven-week history of severe dysphagia. Radiographic examination revealed a stricture just above the cardioesophageal junction. At esophagoscopy, the mucosa over the lesion was intact, but a biopsy from the obstructive lesion at 36 cm from the incisor teeth revealed mucosal lining and muscularis mucosae. Tumor cells characterized by clear cells with hyperchromatic nuclei were present in the muscularis and submucosal layers.

Esophagogastrectomy was carried out, and subsequent pathologic examination confirmed the lesion to be a carcinoid tumor of the esophagus with involvement of the mediastinal nodes. Examination of the urine for 5-HIAA was within normal limits. Six months later the patient died from a coronary occlusion.

It seems probable that the lower esophagus in this case was lined by gastric mucous membrane, although Brenner et al. did not stipulate this. Kulchitsky cells and crypts of Lieberkühn are not found in stratified squamous epithelium, which normally lines the esophagus. The presence of muscular invasion and metastasis in mediastinal lymph nodes indicates that this was a malignant carcinoid tumor.

The Stomach

The rarity of carcinoid tumors of the stomach is indicated by the fact that review of the world literature discloses only 98 cases of gastric carcinoids. In the present series of 135 carcinoid tumors of the gastrointestinal tract, 8 patients with gastric carcinoids were studied clinically and 2 cases were found at autopsy, providing a total of 10 cases of gastric carcinoids.

Upper gastrointestinal bleeding was a prominent feature in the eight clinical cases. In each of these patients, either an ulcer or an ulcerative mass was found. The carcinoid nature of the tumors was diagnosed preoperatively in only two patients with polypoid lesions in whom gastroscopic biopsy provided the correct diagnosis. In the remaining cases the symptoms were usually attributable to coexisting disease, such as peptic ulcer or gastric carcinoma, rather than to the carcinoid tumor per se.

There were associated gastric ulcers in four patients, the carcinoid being found in the base of the ulcer crater. Gastric analysis was performed in three patients, and no hyperchlorhydria was present. Although endoscopy yielded the correct diagnosis in two patients, it only established the diagnosis of associated pathologic processes in the other cases. Barium-contrast studies yielded positive radiologic information but did not indicate the specific nature of the lesion (Figure 23).

All the gastric carcinoids in this series were single and situated in the distal part of the stomach. Multiple primary lesions have, however, been described; Pestana et al. (1963) reported a patient with seven gastric carcinoids. It is noteworthy that in five patients in whom the mass was less than 2 cm in diameter, no overt evidence of malignancy existed either by the presence of invasion of the muscularis or by lymph node metastasis. In five cases, the tumor was 2 cm or larger and overt malignancy was present in all with invasion of the muscularis and the presence of involved lymph nodes in five patients, and evidence of distant metastasis in three patients (see Table 4). The overall incidence of malignancy was thus 50%. In two of the patients, there were associated adenocarcinomas of the stomach, providing a 20% incidence of associated malignant neoplasms (Table 8).

The age of patients with gastric carcinoids ranged between 45 and

55 years, but study of all published cases indicates that the limits of age range from 15 to 89 years. No significant sex differences have been noted.

Treatment consisted of gastric resection in eight patients with wide surgical excision of that segment of the stomach containing the lesion. An analysis of patient survival in the eight patients with gastric carcinoids indicates that four (50%) survived 5 years, and three (43%) survived 10 years (Table 13). Three patients died as a result of massive hepatic involvement by carcinoid tumor.

Significant elevation of urinary 5-HIAA was found in only one of the four patients with hepatic metastases from gastric carcinoids. None of the patients had flushing attacks associated with their carcinoid lesions. One patient with gastric carcinoid had been previously considered in association with a duodenal carcinoid, bronchial carcinoid, and fulminating peptic ulcer disease. Despite

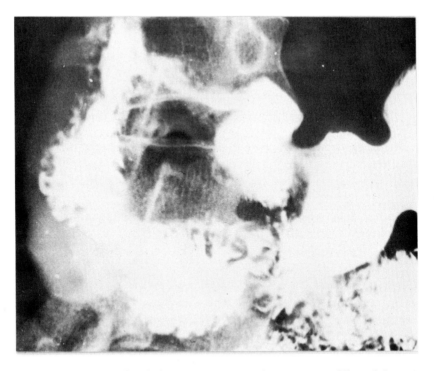

Fig. 23: Barium-meal radiologic examination demonstrates filling defect on greater curvature of stomach due to gastric carcinoid.

Table 13. Survival of 85 Patients with Carcinoid Tumors

| | | 5 Year Data | | | 10 Year Data | | | |
| | | | | | | | | Dead of |
Size	No.	Qualify	Survival	Percent	Qualify	Survival	Percent	Carcinoid
Rectum	37	30	14	46	25	9	35	6
Jejuno-ileum	18	14	8	57	11	5	45	4
Stomach	8	8	4	50	7	3	43	3
Duodenum	8	6	4	66	4	2	50	1
Colon	8	6	2	33	6	2	33	4
Appendix	27	21	17	80	17	13	76	0
Total	106	85	49	58	70	34	49	18

demonstrable lymph node metastases this patient has survived over 16 years. Pack (1964), in discussing unusual tumors of the stomach, reported a patient with gastric carcinoid who continued to do well 27 years after resection.

Von Askanazy (1923) reported the first two cases of gastric carcinoids found at autopsy. A review of gastric carcinoids by Christodoulopoulous and Klotz (1961) described the carcinoid syndrome in association with primary carcinoid tumors of the stomach. They noted that in a collective review of 79 cases, 30 had been discovered at autopsy. In that series, 7 patients had flushing attacks associated with the carcinoid syndrome, which led to a preoperative diagnosis of the gastric carcinoid. Since the review by Christodoulopoulous and Klotz, another 19 cases have been reported, bringing the total reported cases to 98 (Table 14). The addition to this series of 10 patients and 1 patient with gastric carcinoid in association with duodenal and bronchial carcinoids brings the total to 109 patients.

Review of all cases published indicates that the symptoms of gastric carcinoid tumors are nonspecific and are identical with those attributable to carcinoma or ulcer. Epigastric pain is the most frequent symptom, and nausea, vomiting, weight loss, anemia, melena, and hematemesis may be present. The association of any of these symptoms with attacks of flushing or diarrhea should suggest the possibility of a carcinoid tumor. Gastroscopy and biopsy may permit the diagnosis, but barium-meal studies, though demonstrating the presence of a lesion, cannot determine its histologic nature.

Treatment is surgical with adequate resection of the stomach and

Table 14. Gastric Carcinoids

Author	Year	No. Patients	Metastases	Symptoms
Reid	1948	1	0	0
Lattes and Gross	1956	41	11/35	0
Nunes	1958	1	N.C.	0
Wu	1959	1	N.C.	0
Vuborny	1960	1	N.C.	0
Schwandt	1961	1	N.C.	0
Raboni and Maestri	1961	2	N.C.	0
Kantor et al.	1961	2	1	0
Eklof	1961	3	0	0
Christodoulopoulas and Klotz	1961	38	N.C.	6
Vagda and Zulik	1962	1	1	1
Wilson et al.	1963	1	1	0
Pestana et al.	1963	1	0	0
Thompson and Coon	1964	1	1	0
Shorb and McCune	1964	2	1	0
McCraken and Davenport	1965	1	0	0
Total		98	16/45 36%	7

its contained carcinoid tumor. Any nodal metastases should be removed. Wherever possible, metastatic tumorous masses in the liver should be ablated to reduce or prevent the development of the carcinoid syndrome.

The Duodenum

The rarity of duodenal carcinoids is attested to by the fact that only 135 cases of the condition have been published to date (see Table 1).

The present study of 25 patients with duodenal carcinoid distinguishes two separate groups.

1. carcinoids that may cause mechanical effects
2. carcinoid-islet cell tumors

Carcinoids That May Cause Mechanical Effects
Among the 12 patients with carcinoids of the duodenum falling within this category were 8 patients who presented clinically and 4 that were found at autopsy. The tumors were generally small nodules covered by an intact mucosa, and in 10 cases the carcinoid was less than 2 cm in diameter without evidence of overt malignancy. In 2 patients the carcinoid was 2 cm in diameter or larger, and both were considered malignant because of local invasiveness and presence of positive lymph nodes (see Table 5). Distant metastases were present in 1 case. Elevated levels of urinary 5-hydroxyindoleacetic acid were noted in 1 patient with a localized duodenal carcinoid. After its excision the level returned to normal. Carcinoid tumors of the duodenum were asymptomatic in 4 cases found incidentally at autopsy.

The symptoms attributable to this group included upper gastrointestinal bleeding in four patients. In each of these the bleeding was considered to be due to an ulcer or an ulcerative mass. Radiographic features of duodenal obstruction were present in two patients.

The carcinoids were located in the first portion of the duodenum in 10 patients. In 2 patients the tumors were located in the second part of the duodenum, with evidence of associated common bile duct obstruction in 1 patient. In 3 patients, (25%), associated malignant neoplasms were present in the gastrointestinal tract.

In this series of eight clinical cases, four patients survived 5 years, and two patients survived 10 years (Table 13). In only one patient was death attributable to the effects of the carcinoid disease.

A gastroduodenal resection was carried out in six patients in whom a preoperative diagnosis of ulcer or carcinoma had been made. The correct diagnosis only became apparent at subsequent pathologic examination. Pancreaticoduodenectomy was performed for an invasive tumor of the second portion of the duodenum in one case. Local excision of a polypoid tumor of the duodenal bulb was performed via a gastroduodenotomy in one patient in whom the nature of the lesion was diagnosed intraoperatively.

Carcinoid Tumors

A carcinoid polyp of the duodenum that has been seen in recent months has not been included in the integrated clinicopathologic study but merits description. The patient presented with vague dyspeptic symptoms, and barium study demonstrated a duodenal filling defect (Figure 24). At gastroscopy a polypoid lesion was visualized in the first portion of the duodenum, its stalk snared and the tumor removed endoscopically. Histologic examination confirmed this to be a carcinoid tumor. Subsequent gastroscopic examination revealed no evidence of residual tumor, and, accordingly, no further treatment was instituted. The patient is currently being observed.

Review of the literature indicates that among the 135 cases of duodenal carcinoid tumors previously described, many were asymptomatic. Clinical features included duodenal ulcer-like symptoms,

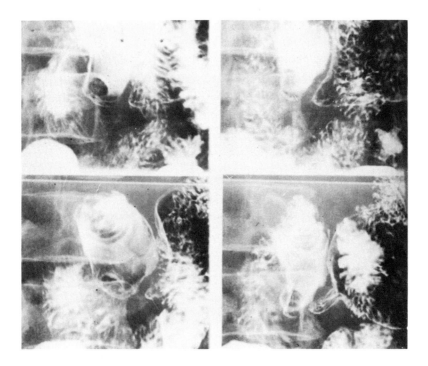

Fig. 24: Barium-meal radiologic examination demonstrates polypoid lesion in the duodenum removed endoscopically and confirmed as a pedunculated carcinoid tumor.

duodenal obstruction, common bile duct obstruction, hemorrhage, and jaundice. The presence of abdominal pain, nausea, vomiting, and diarrhea were also frequently noted. Costello and Aitken (1960) described the development of the carcinoid syndrome in association with a primary duodenal carcinoid.

Carcinoid-islet Cell Tumors
Attention has been drawn to a distinct form of duodenal carcinoid by Nance (1968) and Weichert et al. (1971) who described 13 cases of carcinoid-islet cell tumors of the duodenum at Charity Hospital of New Orleans. I am grateful to Dr. Weichert and Dr. Nance for permission to review these patients.

The term carcinoid-islet cell tumors describes certain duodenal tumors that morphologically and functionally resemble foregut carcinoids and islet cell tumors of the pancreas. Each of these distinct tumors originates from a common neuroectodermal precursor cell that is related to the argentaffin cell. These multipotential precursor cells of neuroectodermal origin have the capacity to develop into peptide-secreting endocrine glands that bud off from the embryonic foregut. Their secretory products, all derived from amino acids, include serotonin, catecholamines, parathormone, gastrin, and insulin (see Table 19).

Radiologicc abnormalities were noted on upper gastrointestinal barium study in these patients. In three patients, filling defects were observed in the first portion of the duodenum. In two patients, there was evidence of a megaduodenum, consistent with changes described in the Zollinger-Ellison syndrome. In six patients there was evidence of duodenal, esophageal, or marginal ulceration.

Gastric analysis was carried out in nine patients and in six over 100 mEq of acid was present in a 12-hour sample of gastric secretion. In two patients the clinical and pathologic features strongly suggested the Zollinger-Ellison syndrome, but the gastric analysis did not confirm it. One patient with 26 mEq acid in 12-hour gastric secretion had a partial gastrectomy which was followed by the development of marginal and esophageal ulcerations requiring total gastrectomy. At reexploration a recurrent tumor was found in the duodenal stump.

In one patient, hyperparathyroidism and nephrocalcinosis occurred in association with a massively bleeding duodenal ulcer. This patient died two days after an emergency gastric resection. Autopsy findings included multiple endocrine adenomatosis with multiple parathyroid and pancreatic-islet cell tumors, as well as a duodenal ulcer.

Five patients demonstrated features of multiple endocrine adenomatosis. One of these patients had a carcinoid-islet cell tumor of the duodenum in association with neurofibromatosis. One patient had a bronchial carcinoid as well as associated gastric and duodenal carcinoids and a schwannoma of the ileum.

Two patients had duodenal tumors with both ulcerogenic and carcinoid features. Each of these patients had a duodenal ulcer. One had a liver metastases associated with elevated 5-HIAA; the other, associated multiple carcinoids of the ileum without measurable increase of serotonin products.

Evidence of malignancy was present in five patients who had lymph node metastases. One patient demonstrated ampullary invasion, and in another the tumor recurred locally after a previous excision. Six of these tumors with metastases or local recurrence were noted to be endocrinologically active. Five of these cases fell within the definition of the Zollinger-Ellison syndrome by virtue of the high gastric acid levels. One patient demonstrated excessive 5-HIAA excretion.

Pathologic examination of this group of tumors demonstrated a size variation from 0.5 to 1.5 cm in diameter. The tumors were circumscribed, nonencapsulated, and limited to the duodenal wall. The tumor was confined to the mucosa and submucosa, with minimal infiltration of the muscularis. Although these tumors were diagnosed histologically as carcinoid tumors and were demonstrated to arise in the mucosa in the region of the bases of the crypts of Lieberkühn, special stains failed to demonstrate beta or argentaffin granules.

Evidence of histologic similarity between carcinoids and islet cell tumors is based upon the impregnation of cytoplasmic granules with silver salts or by clinical or chemical evidence of endocrine function. It is important to be aware that carcinoids may or may not show a positive argentaffin or argyrophil reaction. It is noteworthy that hyperinsulinism, carcinoid syndrome, and gastrointestinal ulceration may occur with either tumor. Shames et al. (1968) have described an insulin-secreting bronchial carcinoid tumor associated with widespread metastases. Van Der Sluys et al. (1964) described a metastasizing islet cell tumor of the pancreas associated with hypoglycemia and the carcinoid syndrome.

Multiple endocrine adenomatosis may present as a familial dysplasia of the neuroectodermal cell system. The common denominator in this syndrome is probably a result of the fact that the neuroectodermal cells migrate to the alimentary tract mucosa where they become argentaffin cells and the islets of Langerhans. A morphologic similarity and functional parallelism has been shown to occur between carcinoid tumors, islet cell tumors, parathyroid adenoma, medullary thyroid carcinoma, pheochromocytoma, paraganglioma, carotid and aortic body tumors, melanoma, oat cell bronchogenic carcinoma, and thymoma. Kaplan et al. (1973) have drawn attention to the fact that carcinoid tumors and medullary carcinomas of the thyroid may contain and secrete calcitonin, serotonin, and prostaglandin E. The association of hyperparathyroidism with carcinoid tumors and medullary carcinoma of the thyroid emphasizes the common secretory potential of these cells.

The Small Intestine

Jejunum and Ileum
During the period of this study, 4611 malignant tumors of the gastrointestinal tract were seen at our institution. There were 87 malignant lesions of the small intestine, providing a 2% incidence. There were 40 patients with adenocarcinoma of the small intestine, 37 with carcinoid tumors and 10 with varying sarcomatous lesions. The slightly greater incidence of adenocarcinoma than carcinoids of the small intestine in our series concurs with the findings of Sethi and Hardin (1969). Rocklin and Longmire (1961) noted, however, that in their series of small intestinal malignant tumors there was a greater incidence of carcinoid tumors than adenocarcinoma.

In the world literature 1032 jejunoileal carcinoid tumors have been described. This locale is second only to the appendix in the frequency with which gastrointestinal carcinoids are found.

Table 15. Symptomatology in Jejunoileal
Carcinoids

Intestinal Obstruction		
Acute	5	12
Chronic	7	
Palpable mass	6	
GI bleeding		2
Asymptomatic		4
Total		18

NOTE: 135 carcinoid tumors of gastrointestinal tract
L.S.U. affiliated hospitals.

In our series, 37 cases of jejunoileal carcinoids were available for
study, represented by 18 clinical patients and 19 autopsy cases. The
latter group represented asymptomatic lesions that were less than
1 cm in diameter.

The ileum provides the most frequent site for the development of
this carcinoid because of the greater number of crypts of Lieberkühn
in this section of the small intestine; 29 such lesions were found in
the ileum; 5, in the jejunum. In 3 cases, the jejunum and ileum were
concurrently the sites of multiple tumors.

The notable feature of small intestinal carcinoid tumors is its
multiplicity with a 40% incidence of multiple carcinoid lesions. In
14 patients there was an associated malignant neoplasm, providing
an incidence of 37%.

Among the 18 patients in whom this condition was discovered
clinically, 4 represented asymptomatic expressions of the disease,
and the other 14 patients manifested clinical features caused by obstruction, bleeding, or the presence of a mass (Table 15). Six patients
were treated by right hemicolectomy with resection of terminal
ileum, and 12 patients underwent appropriate segmental small intestinal resection. It is noteworthy that intraoperative confirmation
of the diagnosis was provided in only 4 cases. In 14 cases, the carcinoid nature of the lesion was diagnosed postoperatively after appropriate pathologic examination. A correct preoperative diagnosis was

considered in 5 patients. Another patient with an ileal carcinoid seen in the past few months but not included in this statistical analysis is worthy of record. The diagnosis was considered preoperatively in a patient with features of chronic partial small-bowel obstruction. A small-intestine barium study demonstrated an area of narrowing (Figure 25). Confirmation of the diagnosis was obtained by selective mesenteric arteriography, which strongly confirmed the probability of the lesion being a carcinoid tumor (Figure 26).

The small intestine is the most common site of malignant and metastasizing carcinoids. Of the 37 cases in this series 23 had evidence of malignancy, as judged by local invasiveness, lymph node involvement, or widespread metastases (see Table 4). It is noteworthy that in a group of 20 cases with lesions less than 1 cm in diameter the incidence of malignancy was 30%. In 12 cases where the lesion was larger than 1 cm but smaller than 2 cm, the features of invasiveness, positive lymph node involvement, or widespread metastases were present. Once the lesion attained a size larger than 2 cm, as it did in 5 cases in this series, hematogenous metastasis were present in all, in addition to local invasions and positive lymph nodes.

Eighteen patients presented with clinical symptoms, and in each the tumors demonstrated malignant characteristics. As lesions became large enough to cause symptoms, the increase in size was associated with local invasion and spread beyond the confines of the bowel.

Significant elevations of urinary 5-hydroxyindoleacetic acid were found in two of seven patients with hepatic metastases from jejuno-ileal carcinoids. These two patients were the only ones in the entire series that manifested the malignant carcinoid syndrome.

Four patients died of the effects of disseminated carcinoid disease. Eight patients of the remaining 14 survived 5 years, providing a 5-year survival rate of 57%. Of 11 patients surviving beyond 5 years, 5 of these (45%) survived 10 years (Table 13).

The average age of patients with small-intestinal carcinoids ranged from 45 to 55 years with no significant sex differences. The condition may occur at any age, and the youngest recorded case was reported by McCartney and Stewart (1959), who described an intussusception due to a jejunal carcinoid in a 4-year-old child.

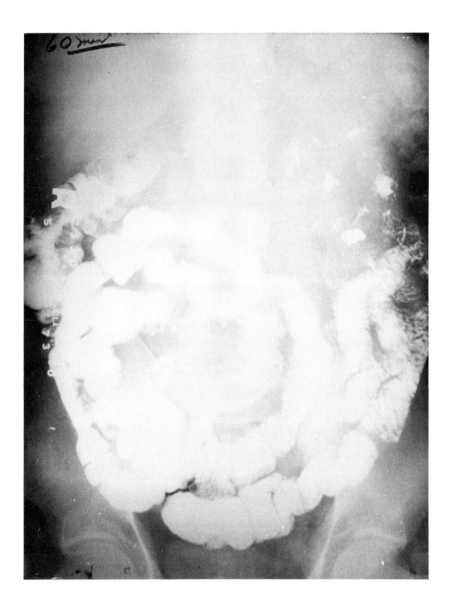

Fig. 25: Barium-meal radiologic examination in patient with persistent colic attributed to subacute intestinal obstruction demonstrates rapid transit and a filling defect in the ileum from a carcinoid tumor.

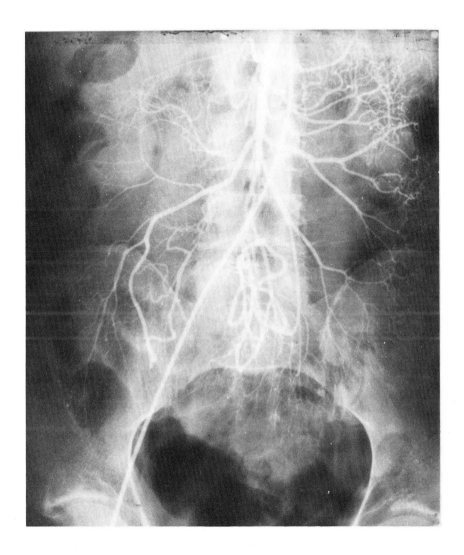

Fig. 26: Selective superior mesenteric arteriography in patient with intestinal barium-filling defect demonstrates narrowing of vessels consistent with changes in carcinoid tumor.

Carcinoid Tumors

Intestinal Obstruction   Among the 12 patients who presented with features of intestinal obstruction were 5 who manifested acute small-bowel obstruction and 7 with chronic obstruction. The obstruction in 1 patient was attributable to a 6 cm tumor situated in the terminal ileum with invasion of the cecum. In 3 patients obstruction was due to intussusception initiated by a carcinoid tumor. In 8 patients, obstruction was attributable to either mesenteric metastases compressing the bowel extrinsically or fibrosis and kinking of the intestine (Figure 27).

Obstruction may thus be caused by:

1. luminal constriction due to intramural spread of the carcinoid tumor
2. serosal fibrosis with interloop adhesions and kinking
3. intussusception
4. intestinal infarction from vascular compression or subadventital fibrosis leading to stricture of the bowel

The radiologic features of intestinal obstruction are nonspecific. They indicate the presence of proximal bowel distention with the

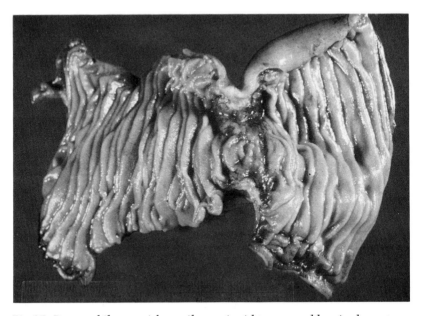

Fig. 27: Resected ileum with sessile carcinoid tumor and luminal construction by desmoplastic reaction.

presence of air and fluid levels. Changes in the contour of the intestinal lumen and in the mucosal pattern are too subtle to permit ready detection. The presence of kinking or buckling of the bowel, intussusception, or a large obstructing mass may suggest that a carcinoid lesion is the source of the obstruction.

Selective arteriography. Reuter and Boijsen (1966) described arteriographic changes in two patients with ileal carcinoid tumors and drew attention to the information provided by selective superior mesenteric artery arteriography. Irregularity and dilatation of the terminal vascular arcades and vas recta may be apparent and attributable to either retraction or the mesentery or subadventitial fibrosis. The presence of a tumor blush may be seen but can be differentiated from carcinoma, which is much less vascular (Figure 28).

Associated clinical features. A palpable abdominal mass was noted in six patients. In one patient the lesion was 2.5 cm in diameter, permitting palpation of the lesion. A 6-cm obstructing tumor situated in the terminal ileum and invading the cecum was clearly palpable in a second patient. In three patients the presence of intussusception provided clearly palpable abdominal masses. In one patient a vague mass was attributable to matting of bowel induced by local fibrosis and kinking.

Massive gastrointestinal bleeding is not a common feature but was encountered in two patients in this series. Exsanguinating small-bowel bleeding has been encountered in another patient in the past few months. Rapid transfusion of 5 units of blood was necessary, and at emergency laparotomy the blood-filled small bowel with serosal tumors was resected. Within the opened segment of the resected bowel, 26 carcinoids were found.

The presence of abdominal symptoms in association with flushing, bronchospasm, or other features of the carcinoid syndrome strongly indicate the probability of a small-intestine carcinoid tumor. Weight loss, constipation, and diarrhea have also been documented as symptoms attributable to small-intestine carcinoid tumors.

Infarction and gangrene of the small intestine may occur as a result of impaired blood supply, but this complication has not been seen in the present series. Anthony (1970) has stressed this important complication of carcinoid tumors resulting from proliferative subadventitial vascular fibrosis.

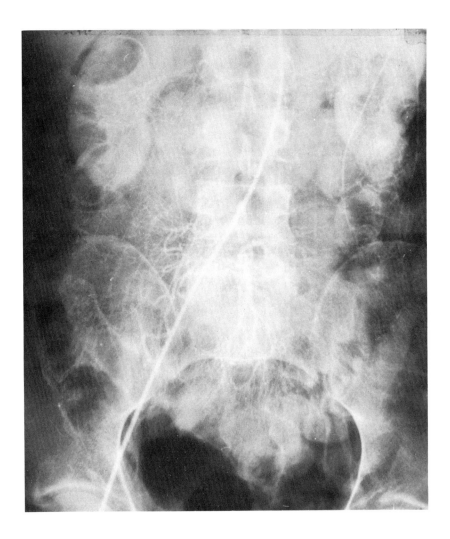

Fig. 28: Delayed film after selective arteriography demonstrated residual tumor blush.

Surgical intervention with small-bowel resection provides the only effective therapy. The mesentery should be resected widely, and any mesenteric metastases should be removed if possible. As much bulk of metastatic liver tumor as necessary should be removed to reduce the production of biochemical substances that may subsequently lead to the carcinoid syndrome.

Meckel's Diverticulum
Although Braxton-Hicks and Kadinsky (1922) reported the presence of an alleged carcinoid tumor in a Meckel's diverticulum, subsequent review of the slides revealed the lesion to represent heterotopic gastric mucosa. In 1926, Stewart and Taylor documented the first carcinoid tumor of a Meckelian diverticulum. In a review of 18 such cases Lechner and Chamblin (1962) described a diverticular carcinoid in a 52-year-old white male. Moertel et al. (1961) reported 5 cases of carcinoid tumors in Meckel's diverticulum, representing the largest series from a single institution.

These lesions are generally asymptomatic, the lesion being a fortuitous finding at surgical exploration or autopsy. Among the clinical effects described are:

1. Partial obstruction around a carcinoid of Meckel's diverticulum with adherance to the abdominal wall.
2. Johnston et al. (1965) reported serious bleeding from an ulcerating carcinoid tumor in Meckel's diverticulum.
3. Symptoms attributable to widespread peritoneal metastasis.
4. Symptoms attributable to the carcinoid syndrome have been described in five cases.

Among the 46 cases of carcinoid tumors of Meckel's diverticulum that have now been reported, the age range has been from 25 to 80 years with an average of 55 years. There has been a marked male preponderance (29 cases). Recurrent peptic ulceration attributable to a carcinoid tumor of Meckel's diverticulum has been described. Excision of the diverticulum with its contained carcinoid tumor led to cure of the ulcer.

Of the published cases 54% of carcinoids in Meckel's diverticulum have been locally invasive, with involvement of the muscular wall. Distant metastases have been noted in 20% of the cases. The liver is the most frequent site of hematogenous spread. A 26% incidence of metastases is similar to that reported for carcinoids of the small intestine in general, which varies from 25 to 38% (Pearson and Fitzgerald, 1949; River et al., 1956).

Wide resection of the diverticulum with several inches of adjacent small bowel on each side of the diverticulum and its mesentery should be performed. If distant metastases are present, they should be resected, and as much metastatic tissue bulk as possible should be removed to prevent the development of the carcinoid syndrome.

Chapter 6

The Colon

During the 22-year period of study of carcinoid tumors of the colon there have been 1640 cases of large intestinal malignant neoplasms. The rarity of colonic carcinoids is reflected in the fact that during this period of time only 10 cases of colonic carcinoid tumors were seen. Two asymptomatic lesions were found at autopsy; six of the eight clinical patients presented with symptoms (Table 16). The symptoms resembled those usually attributable to the more commonly encountered adenocarcinoma. The lesion was clinically palpable in two patients. Four carcinoid tumors were identified preoperatively, one at sigmoidoscopy and three by barium enema. Four tumors were discovered at laparotomy carried out for obstruction in two cases and for perforation of the lesion in one case. One carci-

Table 16. Symptom in Colonic
Carcinoids: 8 Patients

Anemia		1
Weight loss		1
Large bowel obstruction		3
Acute:	2	
Chronic:	1	
Perforation		1
Asymptomatic		2
Total		8

NOTE: 135 carcinoid tumors of gastrointestinal tract L.S.U. affiliated hospitals.

noid tumor of the colon was found fortuitously in the course of an elective cholecystectomy. Except for the one lesion within reach of the sigmoidoscope which permitted biopsy and histologic categorization of the lesion, all the other tumors were considered to be carcinomas until an accurate diagnosis was established at subsequent pathologic examination.

In each situation segmental resection of right or left colon was performed. Evidence of malignancy was present in 9 of the 10 cases studied. There was only 1 case with a lesion less than 1 cm in diameter and this was the only one without any evidence of local invasion or more distant spread. Two lesions were between 1 and 1.9 cm in diameter, and both demonstrated muscular invasion. Metastatic lymph nodes and distant spread were present in one patient.

In seven cases the lesion was 2 cm in diameter or larger, and all demonstrated local invasion and positive lymph node involvement. Six of these cases demonstrated distant hematogenous spread. Overt malignancy was thus present in 90% of the cases (see Table 4).

In five cases, the carcinoid was located in the cecum, in one case it was found in the ascending colon, and in four cases it was situated in the sigmoid colon. Each of the lesions was solitary, so that multiplicity is not a feature of carcinoids of the colon. It is noteworthy that patients with colon carcinoids did not have associated malignant neoplasms. Although seven patients in this group had liver metastases from colon carcinoids, no elevation of urinary 5-HIAA levels was found.

Follow-up of six clinical patients demonstrated two to be alive at the end of 5 years providing a 33% 5-year survival. Two patients who survived 10 years did so despite the fact that there were metastases to the liver. Four patients, i.e., 50% of the clinical group, succumbed to the effects of liver metastases (Table 13).

Six of the patients were male and two were female indicating a male preponderance, and the age range was between 50 and 68 years of age. The youngest recorded patient with a colonic carcinoid was a 20-year-old patient described by Waugh and Snyder (1941).

In the 94 cases of carcinoid tumors of the colon published in the world literature, there is a higher incidence of lesions in the right colon. This fact is reflected in our series of cases. Clinical features attributable to colonic carcinoids are the result of varying degrees of intestinal obstruction with abdominal pain, constipation, occasional diarrhea, nausea, vomiting, weight loss, and malaise. Although bleeding is infrequent, anemia may occur. Barium enema examination will demonstrate a filling defect in the lumen of the colon that is identical with that seen in carcinoma.

Treatment of carcinoids of the colon depends on the site of origin. Right hemicolectomy is indicated in tumors of the ascending colon; transverse colectomy, for lesions of the transverse colon; and left colectomy, for lesions involving the left colon. Colonic resection to prevent obstruction is indicated even if hepatic metastases are present. Frozen-section biopsy of the lesion or of hepatic metastases will guide subsequent treatment, and removal of hepatic tumorous bulk should be carried out whenever feasible. The infrequency of the carcinoid syndrome attributable to colonic lesions may justifiably contraindicate operative removal of hepatic metastases.

The Rectum

From 1948 to 1970, 759 patients with malignant lesions of the rectum were seen at our institutions, and 37 patients with carcinoid tumors of the rectum were seen, providing a 5% incidence. The rectum provided the single most common site for carcinoid tumors in our series. Although symptoms were referable to the rectum in 23 of the 37 patients with rectal carcinoids, the symptoms were caused by carcinoids in only 10 of the patients. Symptoms were attributable to the lesion in 12 patients in whom the rectal carcinoid was 1 cm in diameter or larger (Table 17). None of the 25 patients with

Table 17. Symptoms and Tumor Characteristics of 12 Rectal Carcinoids Larger Than 1 cm in Diameter

Symptoms	No.	Tumor Characteristics
Decreased stool caliber	4	Large proliferative mass
Rectal bleeding	3	Ulcerative lesions
Rectal pain	3	Infiltrating tumor
None	2	Small; no ulcerations or invasions

NOTE: 135 carcinoid tumors of gastrointestinal tract L.S.U. affiliated hospitals.

carcinoid tumors smaller than 1 cm had symptoms attributable to their tumors.

Rectal carcinoids were palpable on digital examination in 22 patients (59%) and were visualized sigmoidoscopically in 34 (92%). In 3 patients with small lesions, the tumors were undetected by either means. A microscopic diagnosis of carcinoid tumor was made on 29 biopsy specimens, 4 of these confirming tentative clinical diagnoses. The carcinoid tumors were described by clinical examiners as firm, smooth, yellowish submucosal nodules. An erroneous microscopic diagnosis of carcinoma was made on the biopsy specimens of 5 patients, and rectal carcinoids were either missed or misdiagnosed in 8 patients (22%).

The presence of rectal pain in association with a carcinoid tumor reflected an infiltrating lesion; in three patients rectal bleeding was due to an ulcerative lesion. The presence of large proliferative masses in four patients led to decreased stool caliber as the dominant symptom.

Variable modes of therapy were applied to the 37 patients with rectal carcinoids (Table 18). Abdominoperineal resections were carried out in 10 patients. In 5 of these patients the original histologic diagnosis had erroneously been adenocarcinoma. These were subsequently reclassified as carcinoid tumors after completion of the operation at formal pathologic examination. In 4 patients the presence of a synchronous concomitant anorectal carcinoma determined the indication for abdominoperineal resection. In only 1 patient was an abdominoperineal resection carried out for the specifically stated purpose of curing a carcinoid tumor of the rectum.

Table 18. Rectal Carcinoid

Treatment

Biopsy	19
Biopsy with fulguration	4
Local excision	1
Anterior resection	1
A-P resection	10
	37

NOTE: 135 carcinoid tumors of gastrointestinal tract L.S.U. affiliated hospitals.

The relationship of carcinoid size to overt evidence of malignancy is indicated by the fact that among 25 patients with lesions smaller than 1 cm in diameter only 3 patients (12%) had overt evidence of malignancy, expressed by local invasion in one case and the presence of lymph node metastases in two. In 6 patients the lesion varied in size from 1 to 1.9 cm in diameter. Of these, features of malignancy were present in 3 patients (50%), manifested by local invasion in 2 and distant metastases in 2. In 6 patients with lesions larger than 2 cm in diameter, overt malignancy was present in 5 patients (83%). Local invasion was present in all 5 patients; lymph node metastases, in 1 patient; and distant metastases, in 4 patients. In the entire series overt malignancy was present in 11 patients (30%) with local invasive features in 8, lymph node metastases in 3, and distant metastases in 6 patients (Table 4).

It is noteworthy that among the 37 patients with rectal carcinoids there were 2 patients with lesions smaller than 1 cm in diameter associated with metastasis to the regional nodes in the absence of muscularis invasion. Study of the patterns of malignant expression provokes an apparent paradox in that a greater incidence of distant metastases than regional metastases were noted. This is attributable to the fact that resection was not performed in several patients in whom distant metastases were discovered at surgical exploration but in whom the status of the regional nodes was not documented.

Carcinoid tumors of the rectum have been classified as malignant whenever either muscular invasion or metastases were found. Consistent with our findings in the entire gastrointestinal tract, the larger the rectal tumor the more probable its malignant propensity (Table 4). Horn (1949), Freund (1957) and Peskin and Orloff (1959) confirmed this relationship of tumor size to the incidence of malignancy.

The middle third of the rectum (i.e., 5–8 cm from the anal verge) provided the locus for 57% of the rectal carcinoids, and 50% of this group demonstrated malignant features; 43% of the carcinoids were situated in the proximal or distal third of the rectum, but malignant features were present in only 7% of this group (Table 7). Multiple rectal carcinoids were found in 3 patients (8%). An associated second primary malignant neoplasm was present in 12 patients (32%).

Six patients with rectal carcinoids had metastases to liver, but only two of these patients had significant elevations of urinary

5-hydroxyindoleacetic acid. Neither of these patients manifested the clinical features of the malignant carcinoid syndrome. Saegesser and Gross (1969) documented the only known case of a rectal carcinoid syndrome associated with elevation of urinary 5-HIAA.

In 30 patients 5-year survival data are available; 14 patients (46%) have survived 5 years. Of the 25 patients available for survey over a 10-year period, 9 (35%) survived 10 years or longer. Six patients died from the effects of their malignant carcinoid disease (Table 13).

Although the rectum provides the most common single locale for carcinoid tumors in our series, it is listed as the third most common site for carcinoid tumors with 500 cases described in the world literature. Dockerty (1963), in a review of carcinoid tumors of the gastrointestinal tract from the Mayo Clinic, noted the rectum to be the most common site of carcinoid tumors; it exceeded the numbers found in the appendix and small bowel, which are generally conceded to be the most common areas involved by carcinoid tumors. From 1941 to 1961, 360,612 microscopic examinations were performed at the Mayo Clinic, and 133 cases of verified rectal carcinoids were found, providing an incidence of 0.04%.

The average age of our patients was in the middle 50s. This is consistent with the findings of Bates (1962) in his review of 253 cases of carcinoid tumors of the rectum. He pointed out that there were no symptoms or signs which were characteristic of this rectal lesion. Although many tumors were asymptomatic, symptoms may include rectal bleeding, changes in bowel habits, and varying degrees of obstruction. The malignant variety of rectal carcinoid may be associated with pain, cachexia, and weight loss.

Since Saltykow (1912) recorded the first description of rectal carcinoid, there have been 706 cases reported.

Gibbs (1963) has suggested that three main histologic varieties of rectal carcinoids should be recognized.

1. The true carcinoid or argentaffinoma. This represents a true carcinoid tumor arising from the Kulchitsky cells.
2. Atypical or nonargentaffin carcinoid.
3. The composite carcinoid.

Gibbs has postulated that the nonargentaffin carcinoids are similar to certain tumors of the lung, pancreas, and gastrointestinal tract and that any differences in growth pattern and staining reactions reflect differing directions of differentiation of the parent epithelium. Morson (1958) suggested that atypical carcinoid tumors arise from the Kulchitsky cells before they are sufficiently differentiated to produce granules. The basiglandular cells of the rectum and the more mature goblet cells have a common embryologic origin from the primitive entoderm. The variable differentiation of the basiglandular cell may explain the occasional histologic similarity between some anaplastic adenocarcinomas of the rectum and malignant atypical carcinoid tumors. Atypical carcinoid tumors have also been found in cases of sacrococcygeal teratomas.

On proctoscopic examination, carcinoids appear as yellowish gray to tan pink and are spherical or lenticular in shape. The small lesions are usually movable, but large tumors tend to become fixed because of infiltration of the muscularis propria of the rectum. Ulceration is rarely seen. Proper histologic identification of carcinoids is possible after hematoxylin and eosin staining. The use of silver impregnation techniques to demonstrate argentaffinity in rectal carcinoids results in false negative reactions.

The rational treatment of rectal carcinoids depends upon the size of the tumor. Local excision or fulguration of lesions under 1 cm in diameter is sufficiently adequate because these lesions are rarely invasive and hardly ever metastasize. In view of the high incidence of local invasiveness and metastasis of these lesions, abdominoperineal resection of the rectum provides the only radical technique available for rectal lesions larger than 2 cm in diameter. Tumors 1 to 2 cms in diameter should be treated by wide local excision as this will cure the majority of these lesions. If subsequent pathological examination demonstrates muscular invasion, then an abdominoperineal resection should be performed.

The Appendix

In the world literature 1686 appendiceal carcinoids have been described, thereby endorsing this vestigial structure as the most frequent site of gastrointestinal carcinoids. Dockerty (1963), on the basis of the Mayo Clinic experience, has suggested that carcinoids arise more frequently in the rectum than elsewhere. Despite this assertion, rectal carcinoids have not been reported as frequently as appendiceal carcinoids. Merling (1838) described the first carcinoid tumor of the appendix, and by 1923 Jackson had found over 300 case reports of this condition in the literature. Collins (1955) reviewed 50,000 appendiceal specimens and noted that 71% of all appendiceal malignancies were represented by carcinoid tumors and only 17% were adenocarcinoma. Moertel et al. (1967) reviewed 34,505 appendectomies at the Mayo Clinic and discovered 109 carcinoid tumors (0.32%). In a review of 26,925 autopsy cases, 7 cases (0.26%) of appendiceal carcinoids were found by these authors.

Only 29 cases of appendiceal carcinoids were found in our series of carcinoid tumors of the gastrointestinal tract. Of this group 27 were noted clinically at the time of appendectomy and 2 cases were found at autopsy. In the 27 patients discovered to have carcinoid tumors of the appendix, 17 underwent appendectomy for acute appendicitis, the operation being an incidental procedure in the remaining 10 patients.

In six cases the tumors were located in the proximal segment of the appendix, all of whom presented with clinical features of acute appendicitis. It is conceivable that the tumor was of etiological importance in causing symptoms due to obstruction of the appendiceal lumen. In the other 21 patients the distal location of the tumor excluded its role in the possible pathogenesis of acute appendicitis, nor could any symptoms be attributed to it. Analysis of the site of appendiceal carcinoids (Table 6) indicates that 2 were situated at the base of the appendix, 4 along its midsection, and 23 at the tip. The carcinoids were single and no evidence of multiplicity was found. Four patients (13%) had associated malignant neoplasms of the gastrointestinal tract. The carcinoid tumor was less than 1 cm in diameter in every instance, and no evidence of nodal or distal metastases were present in any of these cases. In 10 cases, however, overt evidence of malignancy expressed by invasion of the muscularis was present, providing a 34% incidence of malignancy (Table 4).

Of 21 patients with appendicular carcinoids available for analysis of survival, 17 were alive at 5 years, providing an 80% 5-year survival rate. Of these 17, 13 survived 10 years to provide a 76% 10-year survival rate (Table 13). No deaths were attributable to carcinoid disease, and no patients developed evidence of recurrence or metastasis. The average age of the patients with appendicular carcinoids was 26 years, representing a much younger age group than those with carcinoids at other sites. This is consistent with other published series, although cases have been described in children. The youngest patient with a known carcinoid tumor of the appendix was a 5-year-old child reported by Willox (1964).

Appendiceal carcinoids occur more frequently in women than in men. This is attributable to the greater number of pelvic operations performed in females because at the time of the operation incidental appendectomy provides a fortuitous finding of appendiceal carcinoids. Although the carcinoid syndrome has not been described in patients with appendiceal carcinoids, Willox published details of an appendectomy in a 10-year-old girl who suffered flushing for 24 hours prior to appendectomy. At operation a 1 cm carcinoid tumor was found in an otherwise normal appendix without metastasis, and postoperatively no recurrence of flushing occurred. Fabricius (1958) and Markgraf and Dunn (1964) each described a patient with abdominal pain, diarrhea, and flushing found to have metastases from an appendiceal carcinoid producing the carcinoid syndrome. Moertel et al. (1967) have reported a similar case. Prunty and Smith (1965) described a patient who underwent removal of an appendiceal carcinoid and who, nine years later, presented with features of amenorrhea, hirsutism, edema of the face and ankles. She had metastatic carcinoid tumors throughout her abdomen, including the liver and pancreas. The features of Cushing's syndrome were relieved by bilateral adrenalectomy although the adrenals had no metastases.

Appendectomy was the definitive treatment for appendiceal carcinoids in 25 of our patients. One patient underwent a subsequent negative "second look" laparotomy. A right hemicolectomy was performed in 1 patient, but neither residual tumor nor metastasis was found in the resected specimen.

The tumor may generally be recognized at operation or at autopsy as a lesion, which on resection, has a characteristic gray yellow color which generally indicates the correct diagnosis. Microscopic examination demonstrates the cellular morphology to be the same as in carcinoid tumors originating elsewhere in the gastrointestinal tract. The presence of muscular invasion, as noted in 10 patients in our series, is frequently associated with permeation of the mesenteric lymphatic channels but is not associated with nodal involvement or widespread metastasis.

Carcinoid Tumors

The most important consideration regarding the proper management of patients with appendicular carcinoids in the absence of metastasis is whether appendectomy alone is sufficient. An affirmation of this fact represents the orthodox viewpoint, although Knowles et al. (1956) emphasized the importance of searching for lymphatic permeation in the appendiceal specimen before deciding that simple appendectomy was sufficient. Latham et al. (1961) suggested that if appendectomy alone was accepted as the treatment of choice for carcinoid tumors of the appendix subsequent follow-up studies would provide a high incidence of recurrence with widespread metastases. Kantor et al. (1961) considered the presence of a carcinoid at the base of the appendix to be an indication for right hemicolectomy while Ponka and and Antoni (1963) recommended this radical approach for patients who demonstrated subserosal permeation or extension of carcinoid tumor to the mesoappendix or periappendiceal fat. It was for this reason that hemicolectomy was carried out in one of our patients. Review of our experience, however, and comparison with series of patients in whom radical operation was performed confirms that simple appendectomy alone is sufficient therapy unless evidence of nodal involvement is present. The only other indication for right hemicolectomy would be the associated presence of an adenocarcinoma of the right colon. In a long-term review of 110 patients with appendiceal carcinoid tumors treated by appendectomy alone Moertel et al. (1967) noted that, apart from 2 patients who died of unassociated causes, the remaining 108 patients had developed neither recurrence nor metastases at 5-year follow-up. In that series 33 patients were traced 10 years after appendectomy for carcinoid tumor. Although 5 patients had died of unassociated causes, none of the remaining cases had suffered tumor recurrence or had developed metastases.

It would appear that appendectomy alone is sufficient treatment for patients with carcinoid tumors of the appendix in the absence of grossly recognizable evidence of metastasis and in the absence of adenocarcinoma of the right colon. This approach need not be modified even if lymphatic permeation or local muscular invasion is present. A more radical approach may be indicated in the occasional circumstance where the tumor is 2 cm in diameter or larger. This fact would suggest a more rapid and aggressive growth with the im-plication of greater inherent propensity for malignancy, thereby justifying right hemicolectomy.

The Biliary Tract

Since the first report of a carcinoid tumor of the gall bladder by Joel (1929), six further cases have been subsequently reported in the literature, attesting to the rarity of the condition. Bosse (1943) described the only carcinoid of the gall bladder found incidentally at the time of cholecystectomy, all the other cases being found at autopsy. Davies (1959) reported 20-year survival of a patient with extensive hepatic metastases from a primary carcinoid tumor which involved the terminal bile and pancreatic ducts. This lesion probably belongs in the category of periampullary carcinoids rather than carcinoids of the biliary tract.

A study of 189 malignant lesions of the bilary tract and 48 malignant lesions of the ampulla of Vater at our institution provided no instances of bilary tract or ampullary carcinoids.

Analysis of the published cases of bilary tract carcinoids indicates an age incidence ranging from 56 to 71 years of age with no apparent sex difference. In the six cases studied at autopsy, four cases demonstrated local muscular invasion. In two cases in which the tumor was larger than 2 cm in diameter, metastases to the liver were noted.

Among the seven reported cases, Willis (1940) described one patient who had a 6 mm pedunculated carcinoid of the gall bladder as an incidental finding. The patient expired from metastatic carcinoid disease probably attributable to associated multiple carcinoids of the stomach, jejunum, and ileum.

Ampullary Carcinoids

Brunschwig and Childs (1939) described a 44-year-old white female patient with obstructive jaundice due to a periampullary carcinoid tumor amenable to local resection. Since that time seven other cases of primary carcinoid tumors of the ampulla of Vater have been described. The lesions were all treated by local excision except for the case described by Warren and Coyle (1951). They performed a two-stage pancreaticoduodenectomy, but death occurred within five years with metastases to liver, bone, and subcutaneous tissues.

The treatment of carcinoid tumors of the biliary tract naturally depends upon the site of involvement. Cholecystectomy is indicated in the treatment of carcinoids of the gall bladder, but if there is hepatic extension, partial hepatic resection should be performed.

Although local excision may be adequate in carcinoids of the ampullary area less than 1 cm in diameter, serious consideration should be given to radical pancreaticoduodenectomy if larger lesions are encountered.

The Pancreas

Although carcinoids of the gastrointestinal tract were at one time attributed to transformation of ectopic pancreatic tissue, the infrequent incidence of carcinoid tumors of the pancreas emphasizes the probability of a neuroectodermal origin for these tumors. The rarity of the condition is compounded by the histologic similarity between nonbeta adenomas of the pancreas represented by the Zollinger-Ellison syndrome and carcinoid tumors and the ability of the former to secrete not only gastrin but also many hormones including serotonin (Table 19). The spectrum of endocrine abnormalities relating these two conditions has been bridged by atypical cases of

Table 19. Some Examples of Recognized Production of Multiple Hormones by Islet Cell Tumors Including a Gastrin-like Substance

Tumor

Type (?)	Location	No.	Hormones
Islet Cell (usually malignant)	Pancreas (but may have)	1	Gastrin, ACTH, MSH
		1	Gastrin, Glucagon
		3	Gastrin, Insulin (2 of the original 6 presented by Whipple and Frantz)
		1	Gastrin, Serotonin

the Zollinger-Ellison syndrome similar to the carcinoid-islet cell tumors of the duodenum that may have in addition to the pancreatic tumor, tumors of the adrenals, thyroid, and enterochromaffin system.

Pataky et al. (1959) documented the first clear case of carcinoid tumor of the pancreas. Peart et al. (1963) subsequently reported the occurrence of the carcinoid syndrome attributable to a pancreatic duct carcinoid tumor that secreted 5-HT and 5-HTP and that was situated in the tail of the pancreas and associated with metastases to the celiac lymph nodes, the liver, and bones. Bernard et al. (1960) described the simultaneous occurrence of a duodenal carcinoid and a nonbeta cell tumor of the pancreas and emphasized the difficulty of differentiating nonfunctional islet cell tumors of the pancreas from carcinoid tumors. Willis (1940) reported two cases of metastasizing small intestinal carcinoid tumors and suggested that several of the deposits found in the pancreas might be primary tumors. Persaud and Walrond (1971) described a nonfunctioning carcinoid tumor coexistent with a cystadenoma of the pancreas. The carcinoid originated within the wall of the cystadenoma and was characterized microscopically by nests of cells with round nuclei and granular eosinophilic cytoplasm, which provided a positive argentaffin reaction. They were able to demonstrate continuity between the columnar epithelial cells of the cyst wall and the carcinoid cells. Frantz (1959) had previously demonstrated argentaffin cells in the connective tissue of cystadenoma.

The presence of Kulchitsky cells in the efferent pancreatic ducts has been discussed by Williams (1960), who described a patient surviving for 22 years after the diagnosis of an inoperable carcinoid of the pancreas, characterized by a lesion in the head of the pancreas with metastasis to the liver in whom a cholecystojejunostomy provided adequate palliation. Liver biopsy demonstrated tumor cells that were uniform in size and shape with few mitoses and a clear vacuolated cytoplasm which, however, did not stain with the Masson silver technique or the diazo reagent. Although the urinary levels of 5-HIAA were normal, the histologic diagnosis was that of metastasizing carcinoid tumor.

Hallwright and North (1964) described the presence of Cushing's syndrome in association with a carcinoid tumor of the pancreas. Bilateral adrenalectomy relieved the Cushing's syndrome but was followed by skin pigmentation and jaundice. At autopsy, a carcinoid tumor of the pancreas with widespread metastases were found. Although extracts of the tumor yielded ACTH and melanin stimulating hormones, the 5-HIAA urinary levels were normal. The aldehyde fuchsin stain demonstrated no argentaffin properties. However, the histologic appearance of the primary tumor and the cellular arrangement of the lymph node metastasis were typically that of carcinoid tumor.

The carcinoid syndrome has been described in association with pancreatic neoplasms on several occasions. Arnett and Long (1931) reported a patient with a 2-year history of facial cyanosis and telangiectasis associated with edema and diarrhea and the presence of pulmonary stenosis found at autopsy 10 months later. The underlying lesion was described as a pancreatic adenocarcinoma with hepatic secondary deposits. McMullen and Hanson (1958) described the carcinoid syndrome in association with high levels of urinary 5-HIAA attributable to a tumor of the body and head of the pancreas with metastasis to the liver found at autopsy. Dengler (1959) reported the presence of the carcinoid syndrome in a patient who, at postmortem, had a partly differentiated carcinoma of the tail of the pancreas with metastases to the liver, lungs, and lymph nodes. The urine of this patient contained high levels of 5-HIAA as well as small amounts of 5-HT.

These cases, as well as the case described by Peart et al. (1963) were associated with pancreatic neoplasms whose histologic detail varied between adenocarcinoma and carcinoid tumor. The ability of a tumor to secrete serotonin by-products should permit its categorization as a carcinoid tumor rather than an adenocarcinoma.

Chapter 7

Teratomatous Carcinoid Tumors

The Ovary

Since the first report by Stewart et al. (1939) of 2 cases of carcinoid tumors found in ovarian teratomas a further 32 cases have been reviewed and analyzed by Kinley and Penner (1962). Trevenen et al. (1973) reviewed a further 4 cases of primary carcinoids of the ovary and noted that 2 were present in preexisting dermoid cysts and 2 were associated with teratomatous elements. The rarity of the condition is reflected in an analysis of 159 cases of ovarian teratomas at our institutions; 20 of these were malignant and 139 were benign, but not a single case of carcinoid tumor was found.

The ovarian carcinoid arises within a preexisting teratoma in close association with either respiratory or gastrointestinal epithelium and is derived from the argentaffin cells normally found in these tissues. Torvik (1960) described an apparently pure carcinoid tumor of the ovary, but in view of the presence of clusters of ganglion cells a teratoid genesis must be assumed. Although Scully (1970) suggested that the parafollicular cells of teratomatous thyroid tissue provide the cell of origin for ovarian carcinoids, an electron-microscopic study by Toker (1969) confirms that the carcinoid elements arise from Kulchitsky cells in that organ derived from neural crest origin and associated with either gastrointestinal or respiratory epithelial tissue.

Although the condition has been documented in females ranging in age from 21 to 80 years, the majority are 26- to 45-year age group.

The tumor is generally large and clinically palpable at abdominal or pelvic examination. The lesion has always been unilateral and occurs with equal frequency on the right or left side. Bilaterality has not been described. It occurs more frequently as part of a benign cystic teratoma, although it has been found in solid teratomas. Radiologic examination of the abdomen may demonstrate calcification of the tumor.

The tumor is generally solid, smooth, and yellowish white in appearance. Histologically compact clusters and strands of small epithelial cells are found within a collagenous stroma. A fine golden brown pigment is discernible in chromate-fixed tissues, and the Fontana-Masson silver stain demonstrates fine basal or perinuclear argentaffin granules.

The ovarian tumor has varied from 5 to 16 cm in diameter, though Sauer et al. (1958) described a 230-g teratomatous tumor associated with flushing and elevation of urinary 5-HIAA levels. There was a notable drop of 5-HIAA levels to normal after removal of the tumor. Although Douchette and Estes (1965) described two patients with ovarian carcinoid metastases, Holl-Allen (1969) described the only case of an ovarian carcinoid with metastatic disease causing flushing and the carcinoid syndrome. In several other cases the carcinoid syndrome was not associated with metastases and was attributable to the ovarian venous drainage into the systemic circulation.

Oophorectomy or salpingo-oophorectomy provide adequate surgical treatment for the condition. Total hysterosalpingo-oophorectomy is frequently performed if the correct histologic diagnosis has been discovered subsequent to resection.

The Testes

Simon et al. (1954) reported the first testicular carcinoid tumor. Berkheiser (1959) and Sinnatamby et al. (1973) have reported similar cases providing a total of 3 testicular carcinoid tumors in the world literature. In each case the carcinoid tumor occurred in a testicular teratoma. The first two patients were 60 and 50 years old, and the third was a 31-year-old man. Specific staining by the Fontana-Masson technique confirmed the presence of argentaffin granules. The lesion also stained a positive rust red with the diazo method.

In each of the three cases the carcinoid tumor had arisen in a benign cystic teratoma, and, as in ovarian carcinoid tumors, testicular carcinoids are probably derived from gastrointestinal or respiratory teratomatous structures.

Testicular carcinoid tumors may, of course, represent metastases from a primary lesion in the alimentary tract as described by Collins and Pugh (1964). The importance of excluding an intraperitoneal primary tumor has been emphasized by Cope and Newcomb, (1930) who described an epididymal metastasis, and by Kemble (1968), who described a metastatic deposit on the serosal surface of the tunica albuginea. In each instance the primary carcinoid tumor was situated in the small intestine.

In the reported cases of primary testicular carcinoid tumors, the carcinoid component was described as relatively small (less than 1 cm in diameter), representing 20% of the total tumor size.

None of the reported testicular carcinoid tumors were functional and in none was biochemical activity evident. In each the postoperative 5-HIAA levels were noted to be within normal limits, but no preoperative levels had been assayed. Flushing, diarrhea, or other symptoms attributable to the carcinoid syndrome, however, were not present. In the case reported by Kemble (1968) of a primary ileal carcinoid tumor with testicular metastases, orchidectomy did not lead to reduction in the persistently elevated levels of urinary 5-HIAA.

Sacrococcygeal

A single case report by Aparicio et al. (1972) describes a nodular swelling in the retrorectal area involving the sacrum with radiologic evidence of erosion of the lower three pieces of the sacrum and displacement of the rectum to the right. Pathologic examination of the 7-cm cystic mass removed from this area demonstrated a cyst wall composed of poorly cellular fibroblastic tissue and fibrinoid material with a papillary inner layer providing histologic features of an argentaffin tumor with infiltration of the cyst wall and perineural lymphatics. Neither argentaffin nor argyrophil granules were found in silver-stained sections of the tumor, nor was there ultraviolet autofluorescence. Electron-microscopic examination of the tissue, however, demonstrated features which were considered pathogno-monic for carcinoid tumor. Urinary assay for 5-HIAA demonstrated normal levels. In view of the negative argentaffin and argyrophil re-actions the authors consider the carcinoid to be of hindgut origin.

The Breast

A solitary case report by Devitt (1978) of a primary carcinoid of the breast represents a surprising and unusual finding. The tumor was argentaffin positive and was unassociated with any other lesions. The urinary 5-hydroxy indoleacetic acid levels were not elevated.

Chapter 8

The Carcinoid Syndrome

Sir Maurice Cassidy (1931) provided the first recorded reference to what is now understood to be the carcinoid syndrome. Bjork et al. (1952) described the unusual combination of cyanosis with congenital pulmonary stenosis and tricuspid insufficiency. They attributed the valvular abnormalities to a congenital basis, thereby perpetuating the error that Hillman (1943) had made previously in reporting tricuspid stenosis and pulmonary stenosis complicated by carcinoid of the intestine and liver metastases. Isler and Hedinger (1953) and Rosenbaum et al. (1953) associated the presence of valvular heart lesions and flushing with metastatic carcinoid tumors. Thorson et al. (1954) described a series of malignant carcinoid tumors of the small intestine with metastases to the liver associated with valvular disease of the right side of the heart, peripheral vasomotor symptoms, bronchial constriction, and an unusual type of cyanosis. They recognized that this conglomerate symptomatology represented a clinicopathologic entity.

The rarity of the carcinoid syndrome is reflected in a review of the subject by Postlethwait (1966) who found a total of 139 cases of the carcinoid syndrome described in the world literature. In 115 of these cases, the primary carcinoid lesion was located in the small intestine. In the remaining cases, the primary carcinoid tumor had originated in the stomach, the biliary tract, pancreas, and bronchus, as well as in ovarian teratomatous carcinoids. The syndrome has also been described in association with oat cell bronchogenic carcinoma and pancreatic neoplasms whose histologic patterns have frequently been described as that more appropriate to adenocarcinoma than carcinoid tumor.

Although significant elevations of urinary 5-hydroxyindoleacetic acid were found in five patients in our series of carcinoid tumors of the gastrointestinal tract, there were only two patients with clinical manifestations of the malignant carcinoid syndrome. Significant elevations of 5-HIAA were found in one of four patients with hepatic metastases from gastric carcinoids and in two of six patients with rectal carcinoid metastases to the liver. Two of the seven patients with hepatic metastases from jejunoileal carcinoids with elevated levels of urinary 5-HIAA were the only patients in the entire series manifesting the malignant carcinoid syndrome. Elevated levels of urinary 5-HIAA were noted in one patient with a localized duodenal carcinoid, but after local excision of the tumor the 5-HIAA level returned to normal. Elevation of 5-HIAA was not seen in any of the nine patients with liver metastases from duodenal or colonic carcinoids. Twenty-four patients in this series had carcinoid metastases to the liver. Five patients (21%) survived 5 years and four of them survived 10 years. The primary tumors were jejunoileal in three and of colonic origin in two patients. None of the six patients with hepatic metastases from rectal carcinoid survived 5 years. The two patients with the malignant carcinoid syndrome underwent successful partial hepatic resections thereby reducing the frequency and intensity of the flushing episodes.

The carcinoid syndrome is generally associated with hepatomegaly, and metastatic nodules may be clinically palpable. Liver scan may demonstrate filling defects (Figure 29); selective celiac arteriography, vessel displacement or a tumor blush (Figure 30).

Biochemical confirmation of the diagnosis is provided by assay of a 24-hour collection of urine for 5-hydroxyindoleacetic acid with elevation from the normal level of 2–8 mg to over 100 mg. Serum assay will demonstrate elevated levels of 5-hydroxytryptamine.

The intravenous administration of 2 μg of epinephrine will precipitate a typical flush within 90 seconds of injection, providing a confirmatory positive epinephrine provocative test.

Clinical Features

Cutaneous Manifestations: The Flushing Syndrome
Although manifestations such as diarrhea, weight loss, abdominal colic, bronchial constriction, and cardiac manifestations are fre-

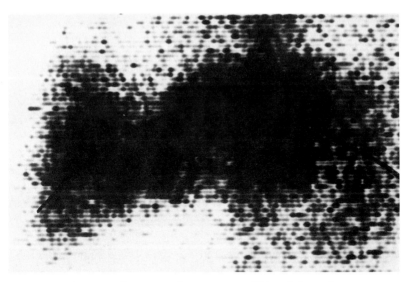

Fig. 29: Technetium liver scan demonstrates filling defects due to metastatic hepatic involvement by carcinoid tumor.

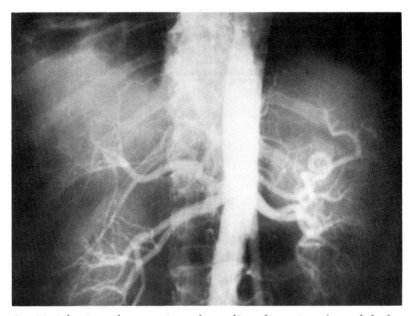

Fig. 30: Selective celiac arteriography outlines distorsion of vessels by hepatic tumorous involvement.

quently associated with the carcinoid syndrome, one of the most striking features of the disorder is the flushing syndrome. This is characterized by the development of a hot flush which commences in the face and spreads to the neck, chest, and extremeties. The flush varies in color from red to orange or may appear as cyanotic patches with spotty areas of pallor. The flushing episodes have been attributed to vasodilatation caused by release of bradykinin into the system. Oates et al. (1964) have demonstrated that increased plasma serotonin is not associated with the flushing episodes but that increased levels of bradykinin may be found in the blood draining the tumor in patients who manifest the flushing episodes and have demonstrated a positive epinephrine provocative test. The flushing episodes may last for only several minutes or in some cases may endure for many hours. In this latter group the flush tends to be of a bluish, cool nature, being associated with vasoconstriction, and frequently is accompanied by wheezing as a result of bronchial constriction. During a flush of this type an increased level of blood serotonin is found draining the tumor (Peart 1966).

The flushing episodes may occur spontaneously or may be provoked by normal activities such as eating, drinking, defecation, and intercourse. It may also be provoked by emotion or physical exertion. Occasionally manipulation of the tumor or palpation of the liver may precipitate a flush. The administration of anesthesia, the insult of a surgical operation, or even the administration of a barium enema may precipitate a severe flushing episode. At such times the patient may experience subjective sensations such as heat and a tightness and tingling of the skin, as well as palpitations, headache, giddiness, and blurring of vision.

Thorson et al. (1958) have described the hemodynamic changes occurring during the attacks and have categorized three stages of the flush.

Stage 1. This stage lasts a matter of 20 to 30 seconds and is associated with burning and flushing of the face with rapid spread into the trunk and limbs. The pulse becomes weak and irregular.

Stage 2. This lasts several minutes once the flush is fully developed and is associated with tachycardia and elevated systolic and pulse pressures.

Stage 3. During this transition stage the flush becomes patchy and may eventually develop a cyanotic hue. The pulse volume becomes weak, and though the systolic pressure is markedly elevated the pulse pressure is lowered.

If skin biopsy is performed at the sites of flushing the capillaries and venules are found to be dilated and congested; the vessel walls, thickened and fibrosed.

Prolonged flushing or repeated episodes of flushing may result in permanent dilatation of the capillaries and venules leading to the development of local telangiectasia and cyanosis. Zarafonetis et al. (1958) have described scleroderma-like fibrotic skin changes attributable to connective tissue proliferation as a response to serotonin.

The flushing syndrome is not always present in carcinoid disease: Waldenstrom and Ljungberg (1955), in a review of 1784 cases of carcinoid tumors, noted that only 75% of patients manifested various degrees of flushing.

In our experience, elevation of 5-HIAA and the presence of hepatic metastases have not always been associated with the carcinoid syndrome in general or the presence of flushing in particular.

The most aggravated forms of flushing are seen in patients with bronchial carcinoids where the episodes may be severe, prolonged, and painful and are often associated with marked facial edema.

Grahame-Smith (1968) has analyzed the flushing patterns and has defined the following clinical categories:

1. A diffuse erythematous flush that is maximal over the face, neck, and upper anterior chest. Milder extension may be observed over the skin of the back, abdomen, and palms. This type of flush usually lasts two to five minutes and occurs paroxismally.
2. A flush that affects the same areas but is of longer duration and is more violaceous. The nose, which is often purple during the flush, frequently retains a permanent cyanotic hue. There are often dilated facial veins and telangiectases associated with congested conjunctivae in these patients.

3. A flush that is usually associated with bronchial carcinoid tumors and endures for several hours or days. The customary flushing areas previously described are red, but not as deeply as in type 1. The rest of the body is more frequently involved, and profuse lacrimation and congestion of the conjunctivae are present. Palpitations are frequently present in association with a fall in the blood pressure. There is swelling of the face, resulting in an exaggeration of the normal facial creases. The salivary glands may become enlarged, and profuse diarrhea may be associated with these episodes.
4. A bright red, patchy flushing interspersed with areas of white pallor that is most frequently seen around the root of the neck. This type of flushing has been associated with gastric carcinoid tumors and has been attributed to excessive histamine production.

Pellagrous Manifestations

As a result of the disturbance in normal usage of tryptophan in the body, pellagra may complicate the clinical picture in carcinoid patients. This is manifested by scaling and pigmentation of the skin of exposed areas associated with glossitis, angular stomatitis, diarrhea, and mental confusion. Under normal circumstances, approximately 1000 mg of tryptophan is present in a normal diet per day and only a small fraction is diverted to protein synthesis, and a smaller fraction is utilized in the 5-HT pathway. Under normal metabolic circumstances, the residue is converted to nicotinic acid in the tissues.

As carcinoids form large amounts of 5-HT, there is reduced niacin production and tryptophan is diverted to serotonin production. The clinical features of pellagra may antedate or be superimposed on the carcinoid syndrome and may be confirmed by the investigations recommended by Sjoerdsma et al. (1957). They noted that during fasting blood tryptophan levels would drop below the normal range of 0.9 to 1.5 mg%, even with high tryptophan ingestion. Estimation of N1-methylnicotinamide (NMN) excretion in the urine is normally 3 to 4 mg per day. In patients with a high urinary 5-HIAA excretion, the N1-methylnicotinamide excretion is reduced in inverse proportion.

The Gastrointestinal System

Although the gastrointestinal system may remain unaffected in the carcinoid syndrome, an analysis of the manifestations of the syndrome by Thorson (1958) has demonstrated that clinical features of intestinal hypermotility occur almost as frequently as flushing (Table 20). Diarrhea may result in 20 to 30 semisolid or watery stools per day, in association with abdominal colic. The gastrointestinal barium meal study will demonstrate a very rapid transit time and the barium may reach the ileocecal valve within 60 minutes. The intestinal hypermotility may result in clinically audible borborygmi. The presence of abdominal pain and increased bowel peristalsis may suggest the presence of bowel obstruction. The manifestations are probably due to excessive production of serotonin and, as shown by Peart and Robertson (1961), serotonin antagonists frequently control the gastrointestinal manifestations.

Table 20. The Incidence of Manifestations of the Carcinoid Syndrome

Total number of cases*	
Male	48
Female	29
Age at presentation	
Male	18–80
Female	33–80
Flushing	74
Intestinal hypermotility	68
Asthma	18
Edema	52
Heart lesions	41
Pellagra-like skin lesions	5
Peptic ulcers	5
Arthralgia	6

* The sex of 2 patients is not reported in the literature.

From Thorson (1958).

Carcinoid Tumors

Symptoms may result from necrosis of hepatic metastases with resulting upper abdominal pain, fever, and leukocytosis.

As peptic ulcer disease may be associated with the carcinoid syndrome or occur alone in association with carcinoid tumors, pain, bleeding, and perforation of the ulcer may provide the presenting clinical features.

The mechanism of abdominal pain in the carcinoid syndrome may be mediated by many causes:

1. pain due to peptic ulceration and its complications
2. intestinal obstruction due to stenosis, intussusception, or tumor
3. abdominal colic due to intestinal hypermotility and diarrhea
4. abdominal pain due to intestinal infarction and necrosis
5. pain due to necrotic degeneration and hemorrhage in hepatic metastases

Diarrhea and rapid intestinal transit may result in excessive fecal fat excretion, leading to malabsorption. Kowlessar et al. (1958) and Nash and Brin (1964) reported that malabsorption may occur in the carcinoid syndrome. Melmon et al. (1963) studied four patients with the malabsorption syndrome by biopsy of the jejunal mucosa, which, however, revealed no abnormalities. Although previous small-bowel resection or lymphatic obstruction by tumor fibrosis may be a causative factor, Melmon et al. (1963) have suggested that the striking improvement in malabsorption after treatment with methysergide, a 5-HT antagonist with a similar molecular structure, implies that 5-HT may be a factor in its causation.

Retroperitoneal fibrosis has been reported as a manifestation of the carcinoid syndrome with involvement of the ureters leading to obstructive renal failure (Bates and Clark, 1963; Hale and Lane-Mitchell, 1964; House and Herman, 1965). It is of some interest that retroperitoneal fibrosis may also occur after the administration of methysergide.

Respiratory System
Bronchoconstrictive effects of 5-HT may lead to wheezing, as well as expiratory stridor and dyspnea. Difficulties in oxygenation may be experienced by the anesthetist if an attack should occur during operative removal of carcinoid tissue.

Mattingly and Sjoerdsma (1956) described the occurrence of asthma and respiratory distress in 20% of their cases. The asthmatic manifestations are generally associated with variable degrees of chronic airway obstruction. The associated wheezing is frequently relieved by isoprenaline aerosol inhalations. Mengel (1965) has indicated that the intravenous administration of methysergide effectively overcomes the bronchial constrictive phenomenon, indicating that 5-HT is the respiratory agent. Thus, the administration of subcutaneous epinephrine is contraindicated in the relief of asthma caused by the carcinoid syndrome because this would precipitate flushing and possibly induce release of bronchoconstrictive agents. Bradykinin and histamine may provide summated effects in the pathogenesis of bronchoconstriction.

Cardiac Lesions
Cardiac involvement, either by virtue of tricuspid insufficiency or pulmonary stenosis, may lead to right heart failure and death. Patients with widespread metastases may survive many years, but patients suffering from the carcinoid syndrome frequently die as a result of the heart lesions rather than as a direct result of the tumor.

The cardiac changes are predominantly those of fibrosis of the valves of the right side of the heart, leading to pulmonary stenosis and tricuspid stenosis or regurgitation. The valvular lesions may result from the high concentration of serotonin, which acts on the valves. As the lung has a high monoamine oxidase content, thereby removing serotonin from the circulating blood, it is rare for the mitral and aortic valves to be affected.

Thorson et al. (1954) reviewed 280 cases of valvular lesions in carcinoid patients. None of the patients were reported to have suffered congenital heart disease, and the lesions in all the cases were described as due to sclerosis and partial fusion of the cusps. None of them developed infundibular membranous stenosis or septal defects. There were no associated atheromatous or arteriosclerotic findings.

Pathologic examination demonstrated the presence of deposits of fibrous tissue on the endocardial surface of the cusps, the chambers of the right side of the heart, and the intima of the great veins and coronary sinus. Plaques of fibrous tissue may also cap the papillary muscles and chordae tendinae. The fibrous tissue deposition leads to constriction of both the tricuspid and pulmonary valves as their leaflets become rigid and fixed. Involvement of the pulmonary valve leads to stenosis, whereas the tricuspid valve may remain fixed in the open position with regurgitation being the predominant lesion.

Only rarely are lesions found on the left side of the heart. When present they are usually combined with involvement of the right side of the heart. McKusick (1956) described the typical carcinoid lesions involving the pulmonary and tricuspid valves in association with lesions of the mitral and aortic valve in a patient with an atrial septal defect. Fischer and Lindeneg (1958) described a similar case.

Roberts and Sjoerdsma (1964) reviewed the cardiac disorders associated with the carcinoid syndrome. Von Bernheimer et al. (1960) described a patient with a nonmetastatic bronchial carcinoid tumor with fibrous plaques on the intima of the pulmonary veins as well as on the mitral and aortic valves, without involvement of the right side of the heart. Three of their nine cases had associated carcinoid fibrous lesions on the left side of the heart, and in these cases the mitral valve was variably involved, and plaques were noted in the left ventricular chamber. All three patients had small intestinal tumors with metastatic spread.

Pathogenesis McDonald et al. (1958) induced the proliferation of collagenous fibrous tissue within the dermis at sites of serotonin injection. Ahmed and Harrison (1964) induced unilateral pneumothorax in rabbits and then administered repeated doses of 5-HT. After several weeks, a thickening developed in the pulmonary arteries but not in the other vessels. The pathologic changes consisted of intimal thickening that progressed to fibroelastosis and variable degrees of medial damage. Foy and Parratt (1960) investigated the effects of the high rate of ingestion of bananas among the Baganda people of Uganda and suggested a correlation between the high serotonin content of their staple diet and the frequency of cardiac conditions such as endomyocardial fibrosis. Similar cardiac involvement has been noted among inhabitants of Nigeria whose diet is equally rich in 5-HT.

Microscopic examination of the cardiac lesion in carcinoid disease demonstrates the local or diffuse deposits of fibrous tissue on the internal elastic lamina. The underlying endothelium, however, is completely normal. The fibrous tissue contains numerous fibro-blasts with much metachromatic substance. Cosh et al. (1959), in an electron-microscopic study of the deposits, noted that the carci-noid plaques were composed of young collagen.

Clinical Features   The presence of precordial systolic murmurs in association with the flushing syndrome and the development of ab-normal jugular venous pulsation should suggest the possibility of carcinoid cardiac disease. Accentuation of the v wave in the jugular venous pulse reflects the presence of tricuspid incompetence, whereas the development of an exaggerated a wave suggests the presence of tricuspid stenosis.

Although pulmonary stenosis and tricuspid incompetence may be marked, it is quite unusual, as emphasized by Roberts and Sjoer-dsma (1964), for right ventricular hypertrophy to be unduly marked. Some cardiomegaly does, however, occur and may be reflected in chest X rays. Electrocardiography will demonstrate the presence of early right ventricular hypertrophy, and cardiac catheterization will confirm the nature of the valvular disorder.

A review of 11 cases of carcinoid heart disease by Waldenstrom (1973) defined the clinicopathologic findings. Subsequent follow-up of the cases led him to conclude that heart disease may be a mani-festation of the carcinoid syndrome with a progressive course of its own even after successful removal of the primary tumor.

Treatment   Without appropriate treatment, cardiac failure ensues and death is the inevitable outcome. As surgical correction is now available for both tricuspid and pulmonary lesions, appropriate clin-ical appraisal is undoubtedly necessary. Carpena et al. (1973) have reported the successful correction of tricuspid and pulmonary valve lesions in a 46-year-old female with the carcinoid syndrome. Their report emphasizes that patients with significant valvular lesions and progressive heart failure from carcinoid heart disease should be considered for surgical treatment.

Miscellaneous Features
Hanna (1965) has described psychosis as part of the carcinoid syn-drome, but very few patients demonstrate psychologic abnormali-

ties despite the importance of 5-HT in cerebral function. This is probably the result of minimal penetration of 5-HT through the blood-brain barrier. Among other clinical features described is edema, which may be the result of cardiac failure or follow vena caval obstruction by a large abdominal mass. Secretion of antidiuretic hormone may lead to sodium retention, aggravating the development of edema. Arthralgia affecting the smaller joints of the hands and feet may simulate rheumatoid arthritis, and very rarely scleroderma may occur.

5-hydroxytryptamine is toxic to the placenta during pregnancy so that premature labor or abortion is almost inevitable in pregnant females who develop the carcinoid syndrome (Reddy et al., 1963).

Techniques for Assay of 5-Hydroxytryptamine

1. Photometric methods. Organic solvents are used to produce a serotonin extract from the tissue protein-free filtrate. It is then allowed to react with 1-nitroso-2-naphthol to produce a chromophore. The serotonin content is then measured photometrically.
2. Spectrophotofluorometry. This provides a more sensitive method for assay of 5-HT. The extracted serotonin is acidfied so that it can fluoresce when activated by ultraviolet light. This technique provides sensitivity to concentration of serotonin lower than 0.04 μg/cc.
3. Biological assay. This is a more cumbersome technique in which the extracted serotonin is treated with acetone and then concentrated. Serotonin can be quantitated to as low as 0.001 μg/cc by its ability to contract the smooth muscle of rat uterus, colon, or stomach.

Measurement of Blood Level 5-HT

1. Serotonin extraction. Serotonin is extracted from the platelets and the result is expressed as micrograms of 5-HT per

10^9 platelets or per cubic centimeter of blood. This provides a very accurate research tool but is too tedious and time-consuming for clinical application.

2. Serum level of 5-HT. After mixing blood with ascorbic acid, it is allowed to clot. During the process of clotting, the platelets release serotonin into the serum while the ascorbic acid prevents the free hemoglobin from oxidizing and destroying it. The separated serum is then frozen and stored for later assay, either by precipitation, concentration, or spectrophotofluoroscopy. The concentration of serotonin in normal serum is 0.1 to 0.3 μg/cc of blood.

3. Plasma level of 5-HT. Heparin is added to the blood sample and the serotonin is released in the plasma. The 5-HT content is measured in a spectrophotofluoroscope for serotonin fluorescence. Normal blood plasma contains 0.1 to 0.2 μg/cc. In the carcinoid syndrome levels may be elevated beyond 0.5 to over 2.5 μg/cc.

Measurement of Urinary 5-HIAA

Examination of the urine for excessive 5-HIAA may be done by screening tests or by paper chromatography of the urine.

Screening tests. Ehrlich's aldehyde reagent combines with 5-HIAA to give a blue color, while the coupling of 5-HIAA with 1-nitroso-2-napthol results in a purple color. These rapidly performed screening tests will register urinary 5-HIAA levels that are elevated above 50 mg per day.

Paper chromatography. Paper chromatography of the urine and staining of the chromatogram with Ehrlich's reagent permits identification of 5-HIAA. If 5-HTP or 5-HT as well as 5-HIAA are apparent on the chromatogram; then a tumor of bronchial or pancreatic origin is probable.

A quantitative estimation of urinary 5-HIAA is carried out by collecting a 24-hour urinary sample, treating it with 1-nitroso-2-napthol to form a chromophore and its 5-HIAA content is quantitated photometrically. In normal individuals, 24-hour urinary collection will contain 2–9 mg but in carcinoid patients, the level may be in the 50–500-mg range.

Carcinoid Tumors

Treatment

Four methods of treatment are available for the carcinoid syndrome:

1. surgical extripation
2. radiotherapy
3. chemotherapy
4. antiserotonin drug therapy

Surgical Therapy
The palliative resection of gross tumorous tissue provides the best method of remedying the symptoms related to the quantitative amount of biochemical hormones produced. The removal of large isolated carcinoid masses from the omentum or liver may provide symptomatic relief for many years. Wilson and Butterick (1959) proposed massive liver resection for control of the severe vasomotor reactions secondary to malignant carcinoid disease. In our series of 24 patients with hepatic metastases, there were 2 with features of the carcinoid syndrome who underwent extensive hepatic resection, with marked amelioration of flushing and diarrhea. A marked reduction in the levels of urinary 5-HIAA reflected the reduced production of biochemical hormones after the extensive removal of tumor-bearing tissue (Figure 31).

Administration of antiserotonin drugs for several days before and during operation will prevent the development of an acute carcinoid crisis that may occur during induction of anesthesia with development of hypotension or bronchoconstriction. Cyclopropane or barbiturates should not be used as these agents may recipitate hypotension. Spinal or epidural anesthesia should also be avoided because of the risk of inducing hypotension. Epinephrine and norepinephrine are contraindicated as their administration may precipitate a provocative release of kinins and 5-HT. During the operative maneuvers it is important to reduce to a minimum the handling of the tumor and thereby prevent excessive liberation of biochemically active hormones.

Radiotherapy
Although an occasional favorable response of carcinoid metastases to radiotherapy has been reported, this mode of therapy is generally

of limited value. In order to be efficacacious, radiotherapy needs to be directed toward the specific lesion in the lung, liver, or abdominal cavity. A prolonged course of radiotherapy was fruitless in one of our patients with a malignant bronchial carcinoid and widespread metastases. Vaeth et al. (1962) have indicated that radiation response has occurred in carcinoids of the rectum, and Mengel (1963) has suggested that radiotherapy may have an adjuvant role in the management of the malignant carcinoid syndrome. Roth (1961) has reported that nodular skin metastases from a carcinoid of the rectum responded well to radiotherapy, reflecting its marked radiosensitivity.

Chemotherapy
Mengel (1965) has reviewed the role of nitrogen mustard, cyclophosphamide, and 5-fluorouracil (5-FU) in the management of carcinoid

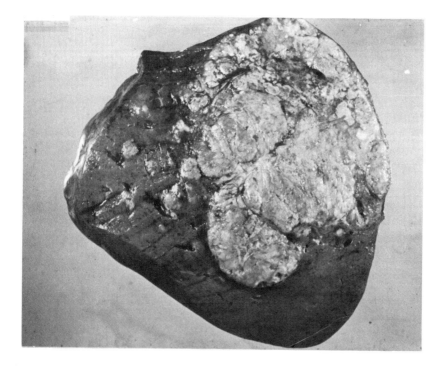

Fig. 31: Photograph of specimen after right hepatic lobectomy. Improvement occurred after removal of hormone-producing tumor.

tumors and the carcinoid syndrome. Although nitrogen mustard has been noted to be occasionally effective, 5-FU has minimal demonstrable antitumor activity. Cyclophosphamide (cytoxan) can produce objective reduction in liver size associated with a transient increase in urinary 5-HIAA excretion and exacerbation of the carcinoid syndrome. This occurs as a result of tumor cell destruction and release of its metabolites, emphasizing the need to pretreat these patients with serotonin antagonists for several days before commencing therapy with alkylating agents.

Legha et al. (1977) recently analyzed their experience with chemotherapy in thirty-two patients with metastatic carcinoid tumor. The effect of 5-FU was contrasted with the effects of nitrosoureas in combination with 5-FU or with cyclophosphamide. In seven patients they utilized Adriamycin in its adriamycin-DNA complex form either alone or in combination with other drugs. Partial response to medication was noted in seven patients, five of whom had received a regimen in which adriamycin was the common denominator. The response to chemotherapy was determined by measurements of 5-HIAA or by changes in tumor size assessed by physical examination, roentgenographic study or radioistopic liver scans.

Moertel et al. (1971) have indicated that streptozotocin causes objective tumor regression in malignant carcinoid disease, but these remissions proved to be short-lived.

It has been suggested that administration of chemotherapeutic substances may markedly increase urinary excretion of 5-HIAA because of the release of pharmacologic mediators from the tumor into the systemic circulation and may precipitate a carcinoid crisis. A similar phenomenon may be precipitated by hepatic artery ligation. The clinical manifestation may be prevented by preliminary administration of cyproheptadine or p-cholorophenlalanine.

Infusion Chemotherapy
Murray-Lyon et al. (1969) suggested that metastatic hepatic carcinoid tumors be treated by ligation of the hepatic artery to induce tumor necrosis. As tumor necrosis may lead to release of vasoactive materials from the tumor, they recommend prior hepatic arterial infusion of 5-FU. After ligation of the hepatic artery, 5-FU is instilled

into a portal vein tributary to destroy any surviving tumor tissue. In two of their patients, remission of symptoms was achieved for five months.

Watkins et al. (1970) have also recommended arterial infusion chemotherapy for the treatment of the disseminated carcinoid disease of the liver. They noted favorable responses utilizing 5-fluorodisoxyuridine (5-FUDR) with favorable objective and subjective responses in four of the six patients treated.

Supportive Management
It is important to support these patients and to hydrate them adequately during episodes of severe diarrhea. A high daily caloric diet should be provided with high fat and carbohydrate content and a reduced (70 g) protein intake. Vitamin supplements should include niacin in those patients excreting large amounts of 5-HIAA.

Antiserotonin Drug Therapy (Table 21)
The administration of pharmacologic agents may be directed to (1) reduce serotonin production, or (2) antagonize serotonin effects after its production.

Inhibition of Serotonin Synthesis
Reduction of tryptophan ingestion from the daily requirement of 250 g to 100 mg is effective for only a few weeks as there is rapid recurrence of clinical and biochemical features aggravated by niacin deficiency.

Parachlorophenylalanine
Parachlorophenylalanine (PCT) inhibits tryptophan hydroxylase, which is necessary for the production of 5-HTP, and thereby prevents the subsequent synthesis of 5-HT. It has no effect on flushing but does relieve diarrhea. The drug is administered in doses of up to 4 g per day and has demonstrable efficacy in 80% of patients. It also reduces the level of urinary 5-HIAA (Engelman et al., 1967).

Blockade of the Conversion of 5-HTP to 5-HT
This step requires cofactor pyridoxine and the enzyme decarboxylase. Pyridoxine deficiency may be induced by administration of

Table 21. Carcinoid Syndrome Metabolic Pathway†

Pharmaceutical Antagonists	Metabolic Pathway	
	Tryptophan	
Parachlorphenylalanine		
Methysergide (Sansert)	Tryptophan	
Cyproheptidine (Periactin)	5-hydroxylase	
	5-Hydroxytryptophan	
Methyldopa	aromatic L-amino acid decarboxylase	Tumor
	5-Hydroxytryptamine	
Chlorpromazine	Monoamine oxidase	
Corticosteroids		
		Blood
INH	5-Hydroxyindole Acetaldehyde	
Heparin	aldehyde	
Regitine	dehydragenase	
	5-Hydroxyindoleacetic Acid	Urine
5-FU		
Cyclophosphamide	Indoleacetic Aicd	

NOTE: 135 carcinoid tumors of gastrointestinal tract L.S.U. affiliated hospitals.

pyridoxine inhibitors such as desoxypyridoxine, or pyridine-binding agents, which increase its excretion. Mengel (1965) utilized isonicotinic acid hydrazine. These agents have not been materially effective in controlling the symptoms of the carcinoid syndrome and have undesirable side effects.

Decarboxylase Inhibitors
Alpha-methyl-dopa was the first agent utilized to inhibit the synthesis of 5-HT by blocking the conversion of 5-HTP to 5-HT. It is generally ineffective in relieving symptoms, it fails to reduce the 5-HIAA urinary level, and it produces many undesirable side effects.

Mengel (1965) suggested that these drugs may have a role in patients with gastric tumors that secrete large amounts of 5-HTP.

Miscellaneous Drugs

Melmon et al. (1965) have demonstrated that trasylol, a commercially prepared kallikrein inhibitor, can inhibit the synthesis of carcinoid tumor kallikrein in vitro. Infusion of large amounts of trasylol have, however, failed to provide any therapeutic benefits.

Beta-adrenergic blockade may relieve the effects of catecholamines released by the stimulatory effect of emotion, diet, exercise, and alcohol. Phenoxybenzamine may be administered three times a day. A daily dosage of 10–20 mg may substantially relieve the severity of flushing attacks. Unfortunately this drug has side effects such as dizziness and nasal stuffiness which tend to limit its use. Ludwig et al. (1968) suggested that the beta-blocking agent propranolol might be equally effective in reducing the flushing episodes.

Chlorpromazine, an alpha-adrenergic blocker, has antikinin effects and may control flushing. It may also be administered prior to the introduction of chemotherapy.

Inhibition of Serotonin Activity

Mengel (1965) suggested that a combination of drugs tends to be more effective than any one drug alone. He noted that in some patients with the carcinoid syndrome only the diarrhea is relieved, whereas in others either the flushes or the bronchospasm is ameliorated.

The specific serotonin antagonists available are:

1. Methysergide maleate (Sansert). This serotonin inhibitor is a potent antagonist of 5-HT and is the most effective of all the available drugs. It is administered in divided doses to a total of 3–8 mg per day and exerts its maximal benefit in the control of diarrhea. This drug has frequently been used in the treatment of migraine. Side effects with its prolonged usage include vascular spasm and the development of retroperitoneal fibrosis.

2. Cyproheptadine (Periactin). This 5-HT antagonist is occa-

sionally effective in controlling diarrhea and less frequently may reduce the intensity of flushing.

3. 1-*N*-Methylpiperidyl-4-3-phenylbenzyl-pyrazolone-5 (KB-95).

Nonspecific Measures

Prednisone in a dosage of 20 mg daily may relieve the flushing caused by bronchial carcinoids. It is also effective in relieving the hyperdynamic cardiac state as well as the facial edema, diarrhea, and general distress associated with bronchial carcinoids. It is, however, totally ineffective in controlling the flush or the diarrhea induced by gastrointestinal carcinoid tumors.

Summary

This clinicopathologic study of carcinoid tumors indicates that carcinoids develop in the submucosa even though they originate in the mucosa. The tumor is composed of small cells that are uniform in size and exist in several variant patterns. Neither cellular morphology nor histologic architecture can be used to distinguish relative degrees of benignity or malignancy.

Extension of the tumor usually occurs in a horizontal fashion within the submucosa, and the tumor tends to grow away from the lumen. The more aggressive lesions penetrate the wall of the viscus of origin subsequently invading the mesentery, parietal peritoneum, and adjacent organs. Metastases, when present, usually occur in the regional lymph nodes and liver, and less frequently in other distant sites such as lung, brain, and bone.

McDonald (1956) first proposed an index of malignancy exclusive of discernible metastases and suggested that carcinoids should be reported in terms of invasiveness. Peskin and Orloff (1959) and Orloff (1971) demonstrated a striking correlation between size and malignant behaviour in rectal carcinoids. Our study confirms the relationship between size and invasiveness, on the one hand, and the occurrence of metastases, on the other, for all extra-appendiceal carcinoids. Our data further indicates that the aggressiveness of these extra-appendiceal tumors in the 1–2 cm range approaches or equals that of the larger lesions.

The relationship between carcinoid structure and function has been enunciated by Williams and Sandler (1963) and permits a categorization of all carcinoids.

1. Foregut derivatives: stomach, duodenum, pancreas, biliary tract, and bronchus. The cells 180-200 μ in size are regularly shaped, have a trabecular arrangement, and contain round granules. The

cells cannot be stained with metallic silver unless a reducing agent is present, providing an argyrophilic reaction.

2. Midgut derivatives: jejunum, ileum, and right colon. The cells are pleomorphic and vary in size from $75-500$ μ. They are arranged in nests separated by delicate connective tissue stroma. They demonstrate both argentaffin and argyrophilic characteristics.

3. Hindgut derivatives: the left colon and rectum. The cells, $165-235$ μ in diameter, are arranged in trabecular form and contain round regular granules. They do not stain with silver. Variant manifestations may be associated with the carcinoid syndrome due to tumors derived from the stomach or bronchi. As these tumors secrete very little 5-HT but large quantities of 5-HTP, assay of urine may demonstrate high levels of 5-HTP and 5-HIAA.

Gastric carcinoids tend to metastasize to the peritoneal cavity and lead to the development of a bright red, generalized flush. Bronchial tumors metastasize to bones and skin and the carcinoid flush is prolonged, painful, and frequently associated with facial edema. Metastases from small-intestinal carcinoids frequently produce the carcinoid syndrome since these tumors contain large amounts of serotonin, which is present in the blood system. Urinary 5-HIAA is high and flushes are frequently present in this syndrome. Metastases are generally confined to the peritoneal cavity.

Carcinoids of the hindgut are rarely associated with metabolic disturbances or flushes and are not associated with elevations of serum 5-HT or 5-HTP or urinary 5-HIAA. Metastatic spread occurs in bone, skin, and structures within the peritoneal cavity.

Carcinoid tumors of the stomach, duodenum, appendix, and rectum may be asymptomatic or symptoms may be related to associated diseases. Carcinoids of the large and small intestine usually provide symptoms that may be long-standing or dramatic and acute. Symptoms of colon carcinoids are indistinguishable from those of adenocarcinoma, and carcinoids beyond the reach of the sigmoidoscope are usually diagnosed as carcinoma by barium enema or laparotomy.

Symptomatic jejunoileal carcinoids cause acute or chronic intestinal obstruction. A small intramural jejunal or ileal carcinoid does not readily obstruct the bowel lumen but may serve as a source of an intussusception. More frequently the bowel may be kinked by neoplastic or fibrotic distortion of the mesentery, the primary tumor itself being inconspicuous. Multicentric tumors are frequently found in the small intestine and occasionally in patients with rectal lesions. It is not a feature of carcinoids in other locations.

The high incidence of associated malignant neoplasms in patients with carcinoid tumors was first described by Pearson and Fitzgerald (1944) who found a 23% incidence in their autopsy series. This association in our series has been found to be more frequent than previously reported. A further interesting finding in our series was the fact that the associated malignant disease was responsible for more deaths than the carcinoid.

Analysis of survival data indicates that carcinoid tumors of the appendix carry an excellent prognosis, and the outlook is poorest for patients with colonic carcinoids. The prognosis for patients with other gastrointestinal carcinoids is reasonably good, the survival rate in our series varying from 46% to 66%.

Long-term survival can be expected in patients with gastrointestinal carcinoids, as well as in patients with carcinoids of the bronchus, even in the presence of recurrence or metastases. Thus the role of palliative resection cannot be underestimated. Wilson and Butterick (1959) first reported the benefits of palliative hepatic resection for symptomatic metastatic carcinoids, and of our 24 patients with hepatic metastases, 21% survived five years. Two of these patients had undergone successful hepatic resection.

A review of 172 patients with carcinoid tumors of the gastrointestinal tract and the respiratory system provides clinical and pathological data that permits valid comparison between our experience and the collected world experience.

Among 28 patients with bronchial adenomas, 24 (86%) were of the carcinoid type and represent an incidence of 0.6% of all primary lung tumors seen in our institutions. There is a slightly greater female preponderance and a greater incidence in the right bronchopulmonary tree than the left. Symptoms may exist for many years before the condition is diagnosed, and prolonged survival for many years occurred even in the absence of surgical treatment. Although pneumonectomy was performed in several patients, lobectomy was generally curative.

The commonest site for carcinoids of the gastrointestinal tract are the appendix, jejunoileum, and rectum. Regardless of location, gastrointestinal carcinoids smaller than 1 cm in diameter only rarely demonstrate evidence of malignant potential. Lesions in the 1–1.9-cm range demonstrate malignant potential to a variable degree while tumors 2 cm or larger are invariably invasive, metastatic, or both. All gastrointestinal carcinoids, except those of the appendix, enlarge, invade, and metastasize predictably, if sufficient time elapses.

Carcinoids of the stomach, duodenum, appendix, and rectum may be asymptomatic, and many are discovered coincidentally at operation, at autopsy, or at proctoscopy prior to attaining sufficient size to cause symptoms.

Carcinoids of the jejunum and ileum may cause intestinal obstruction while still small, but usually after attaining a size of 2 cm or larger.

Carcinoids of the duodenum may be of two types. The first type is similar to those occurring elsewhere in the gastrointestinal tract; the second category is represented by carcinoid-islet cell tumors that morphologically and functionally have features of foregut carcinoids and islet cell tumors of the pancreas.

These tumors are frequently associated with peptic ulceration and often demonstrate features of multiple endocrine adenomatosis. The clinical and pathologic features may be very similar to the Zollinger-Ellison syndrome.

With the exception of colonic carcinoids, the gastrointestinal carcinoid carries a better prognosis than adenocarcinoma. The 5-year survival rates vary from 45 to 100%. Even in the presence of distant metastases, 5- and 10-year survival occurs in a significant number of patients. Rectal carcinoids that have given rise to distant metastases, however, are almost uniformly fatal in a relatively short period of time. The frequent concomitant presence of associated malignant disease accounts for as many or more deaths in these patients than the carcinoids themselves.

The occasional presence of carcinoid elements in teratomatous tumors of the ovary, testicle, and sacrococcygeal repair was considered.

The malignant carcinoid syndrome is reviewed in the light of its biochemical and endocrinologic effects. Techniques used in assaying carcinoid hormones are considered and the therapeutic modalities available for control of the carcinoid syndrome are described.

Acknowledgments

My thanks to Drs. J. Morgan and C. Hearn, surgical residents who helped in the review of patients with carcinoids of the gastrointestinal tract, and to Dr. Lamberty, who aided me in the electron-microscopic studies. I am grateful to the secretarial staffs in the Tumor Registries of Charity Hospital and the Veteran's Administration Hospital of New Orleans for their help in gathering the statistical data. I wish to express my appreciation to the Art Department of the Louisiana State University Medical School for the illustrative work and to Mrs. Mary Engelhardt and Mrs. Mildred Boatner for their secretarial services. I wish to thank my colleague, Dr. Ernest Cohen, for providing the photograph in Figure 5. The editor of Acta Med. Scand. very generously permitted reproduction of Table 20.

Appendix

Gastric Carcinoids: 10

Hospital Number	Age	Sex	Race
54-136797	38	F	B
60-349145	60	F	W
69-215697	26	M	B
71-279515	58	M	W
50-419715	80	F	B
54-148511	60	M	B
55-178913	51	M	B
59-313448	65	F	B
60-340755	38	M	B
62-8588	32	F	B

Duodenal Carcinoids: 25

Conventional: 12

Hospital Number	Age	Sex	Race
49-306506	36	F	B
53-106040	69	M	B
54-149272	78	F	B
63-35553	53	F	B
64-62167	56	M	B
69-206207	68	M	B
72-284732	77	M	B
43-89405	54	M	B
64-81187	49	M	B

A2097	40	M	B
A1421	69	M	B
A191	41	M	B

Carcinoid-Islet Cell Tumors: 13

49-397297	27	M	B
60-340755	40	M	B
54-153940	51	M	B
66-130113	53	M	B
57-275069	33	M	B
66-132639	43	F	B
66-116476	44	F	B
53-121718	35	M	B
67-153982	49	M	B
A1950	65	M	B
435-60-5448	34	F	B
65-116476	44	F	B
437-07-8167	40	M	B

Jejunoileal Carcinoids: 37

Hospital Number	Age	Sex	Race
48-299517	65	M	B
49-360266	44	F	B
49-377805	42	F	B
50-424137	42	M	B
51-21332	57	F	W
51-29700	59	M	B
54-146907	64	M	B
55-184813	66	F	B
56-233250	74	M	B
57-265697	75	M	B
60-364858	39	F	B
62-8255	70	M	B
62-24681	50	F	B
65-99090	65	F	B

65-99599	68	M	B
65-103869	65	F	B
66-118831	78	M	W
67-170710	66	M	B
69-204941	65	M	B
69-212055	54	M	W
44-139319	61	F	B
45-192817	69	F	B
47-270279	50	M	B
52-78616	64	M	B
52-78780	59	M	W
53-105870	74	M	W
54-133385	74	M	B
56-230491	30	M	B
57-259046	74	M	W
62-22766	87	F	W
62-26536	72	F	B
65-117886	58	M	B
69-219616	49	M	B
57-257143	60	F	W
A5300	43	M	B
A13843	50	M	B
A14620	56	M	B

Carcinoids of the Colon: 10

Hospital Number	Age	Sex	Race
49-355037	52	F	W
51-42590	39	F	W
57-268998	67	M	W
58-295246	55	F	B
62-24865	57	F	W
63-57427	80	F	B
50-445969	63	F	B
66-124699	56	M	B
59-322654	69	F	B
11230	66	M	W

Rectal Carcinoids: 37

Hospital Number	Age	Sex	Race
42-447	43	F	B
42-2814	82	F	W
44-161657	50	M	B
49-399154	65	M	B
52-46644	69	M	B
53-92588	47	F	B
54-132277	62	M	B
54-133154	31	F	B
57-260611	45	M	W
61-394913	59	F	B
62-6604	64	F	B
62-8518	58	F	B
62-10865	63	F	W
62-28339	55	F	W
63-41913	33	F	B
63-50717	64	M	W
65-105859	64	M	W
66-145217	50	F	B
67-162194	61	F	B
68-181435	41	F	B
69-220642	58	F	B
69-225851	41	F	B
71-280352	67	M	B
46-204458	61	F	B
60-340942	60	F	B
63-35255	63	F	B
63-47504	20	M	B
66-121803	63	F	W
70-239379	53	F	B
73-319480	42	F	B
51-40413	64	F	B
58-300084	31	M	B
A7843	66	M	B
A8537	63	M	W

A6140	49	M	W
A1431	43	M	W
A14701	66	M	B

Carcinoids of Appendix: 29

Hospital Number	Age	Sex	Race
44-147380	66	F	B
48-338434	49	M	W
49-373946	14	F	B
53-91774	32	F	B
43-106607	39	F	B
53-111532	39	M	B
53-116444	11	F	W
54-165055	17	F	B
56-208837	7	M	W
57-249357	17	M	W
59-335681	14	F	W
63-37981	43	F	B
63-38267	37	F	B
63-5330	23	F	W
64-61279	30	F	B
64-87578	24	M	B
65-89794	22	F	B
65-98195	64	F	B
67-151376	21	F	B
70-244537	60	F	B
47-281173	46	F	B
50-438789	36	F	B
51-8182	35	M	B
51-23201	14	F	W
54-147947	14	M	B
60-351194	8	F	B
62-1423	28	M	B
64-67613	9	M	W
72-289530	39	F	W

Bronchial Adenomas: 28
Carcinoids: 24

Hospital Number	Age	Sex	Race
62-3042	54	F	W
62-14019	42	M	B
64-85185	47	F	B
65-108208	30	M	B
67-159383	62	F	W
69-202063	70	M	B
48-304666	48	F	B
49-350826	44	F	B
57-253491	45	F	W
59-314878	21	F	W
59-331128	22	F	W
61-385758	19	F	W
64-61238	50	F	W
42-04869	66	M	B
43-4869	60	M	B
48-269969	58	M	W
53-93044	58	F	W
427-10-7472	57	M	B
437-32-9500	40	F	W
A15656	64	M	W
428-03-1838	65	F	B
462-40-7980	29	M	B
A3547	64	M	W
A1252	49	M	B

Noncarcinoids: 4

52-62050	58	F	B
46-241698	66	F	W
69-282672	56	M	B
49-375797	57	M	B

References

Adamson, J. E., and Postlethwait, R. W. Carcinoid Tumors Of The Gastrointestinal Tract. Ann. Surg. 148:239, 1958.

Ahmed, F. S., and Harrison, C. V. Morphological Effects of Serotonin on Pulmonary Arteries. An Experimental Study In Rabbits. J. Path. Bact. 87:324, 1964.

Altman, H. W. and Schutz, W. Ueber Ein Knochenhaltiges Bronchuscarcinoid. Beitrage Pathologischen Anatomie Und Pathologie. 120:455, 1968.

Anderson, J. A., Ziegler, M. R., and Doeden, D. Banana Feedings And Urinary Excretion Of 5-Hydroxyindoleacetic Acid. Science. 127:236, 1958.

Anthony, P. P., and Drury, R. A. B. Elastic Vascular Sclerosis Of Mesenteric Blood Vessels In Argentaffin Carcinoma. J. Clin. Path. 23:110, 1970.

Anthony, P. P., Gangrene Of The Small Intestine. A complication of argentaffin carcinoma. Brit. J. Surg. 57:118, 1970.

Aparicio, S. R., Cowen, P. N., and Croft, C. B. Argentaffin Carcinoma Arising In A Sacrococcygeal Teratoma. J. Path. 107:49, 1972.

Arnett, J. H., and Long, C. F. A Case Of Congenital Stenosis Of The Pulmonary Valve With Late Onset Of Cyanosis. Death from carcinoma of the pancreas. Amer. J. Med. Sci. 182:212, 1931.

Aschoff, L. E. ed. Pathologische Anatomie, ein Lehrbuch fur Studierende und Arzte. 3rd Auff. Jena. Germany. Verlag Von Gustav Fischer p. 831, 1911.

Ashworth, C. T., and Wallace, S. A. Unusual Locations Of Carcinoid Tumors. Arch. Path. 32:272, 1941.

Askanazy, Von M. ZurPathogenese Der Magenkrebse Und Uber Ihten Gelegentlichen Ursprung Aus Angebrorenen Epithelialen Keimen In Der Magenwand. Dtsch. Med. Wochenscht., 49:49, 1923.

Azzopardi, J. G., and Bellan, A. R. Carcinoid Syndrome And Oat Cell Carcinoma Of The Bronchus. Thorax. 20:393, 1965.

Barnes, T. G. Argentaffinoma (carcinoid) Of The Gallbladder. A case report. Surgery. 32:723, 1952.

Bates, H. R. Jr. Carcinoid Tumors Of The Rectum. Dis. Colon Rectum. 5:270, 1962.

Bates, H. R. and Clark, R. F. Observations On The Pathogenesis Of Carcinoid Heart Disease And The Tanning Of Fluorescent Fibrin By 5-hydroxytryptamine And Caeroplasmia. Am. J. Clin. Path. 39:46, 1963.

Bates, H. R. and Belter, L. F. Composite Carcinoid Tumor (argentaffinoma-adenocarcinoma) Of The Colon. Report of two cases. Dis. Colon Rectum. 10:467, 1967.

Becker, F. P. Argentaffinoma Of Meckel's Diverticulum And Adjacent Ileum. Gastroenterology. 38:646, 1960.

Beger, A. Ein Fall Von Krebs des Wurmfort Satzes. Berl. Klin. Wochenschr. 19:616, 1882.

Benditt, E. P., and Rowley, D. A. Antagonism Of 5-hydroxytryptamine By Chlorpromazine. Science. 123:24, 1956.

Bensch, K. G., Gordon, G. B., and Miller, L. R. Electronmicroscopic And Biochemical Studies On The Bronchial Carcinoid Tumor. Cancer. 18:592, 1965.

Bernard, C., Gerber, A., and Shields, T. W. Simultaneous Duodenal Carcinoid And Non-beta Cell Tumor Of The Pancreas. Arch. Surg. 81:379, 1960.

Berkheiser, S. W. Carcinoid Tumor Of The Testis Occurring In A Cystic Teratoma Of The Testis. J. Urol. 82:352, 1959.

Bjorck, G., Axen, O., and Thorson, A. Unusual Cyanosis In A Boy With Congenital Pulmonary Stenosis And Tricuspid Insufficiency. Fatal outcome after angiocardiography. Am. Heart. J. 44:143, 1952.

Blackwell, W. J. Argentaffin Carcinoma Arising In An Ovarian Dermoid Cyst. Am. J. Obst. and Gynec. 51:576, 1946.

Bosse, M. D. Carcinoid Tumor Of The Gallbladder. Arch. Pathol. 35:898, 1943.

Braxton-Hicks, J. A. and Kadinsky, S. Carcinoid Tumor Of A Meckel's Diverticulum. Lancet. 2:70, 1922.

Brenner, S., Heimlich, H., and Widman, M. Carcinoid Of Esophagus. N. Y. State J. Med. 69:1337, 1969.

Brookes, V. S., Waterhouse, J. A. H., and Powell, D. J. Malignant Lesions Of The Small Intestine. Brit. J. Surg. 55:405, 1968.

Brown, H., and Lane, M. Cushing's And Malignant Carcinoid Syndromes From Ovarian Neoplasms. Arch. Intern. Med. 115:490, 1965.

Brunschwig, A., and Childs, A. Resection Of Carcinoma (carcinoids) Of The Infrapapillary Portion Of The Duodenum Involving The Ampulla Of Vater. Am. J. Surg. 45:320, 1939.

Burcharth, F., and Axelson, C. Bronchial Adenomas. Thorax. 27:442, 1972.

Burkhardt, F. Zur Lehre Der Kleinen Dünndarmkatzinone. Frankf. Ztschr. F. Path. 3:593, 1909.

Buse, J., Buse, M. G., and Roberts, W. J. Eosinophilic Adenoma Of The Pituitary And Carcinoid Tumor Of The Recto-sigmoid Area. J. Clin. Endocr. 21:735, 1961.

Carpena, C., Kay, J. H., Mendez, H. M., Redington, J. V., Zubiate, P., and Zucker, R. Surgery In Carcinoid Heart Disease. Amer. J. Cardiol. 32:229, 1973.

Cassidy, M. A. Postmortem Findings In Case Shown On October 10, 1930 As One Of Abdominal Carcinomatosis With Probable Adrenal Involvement. Proc. Roy. Soc. Med. 24:920, 1931.

Chatterjee, K., and Heather, J. G. Carcinoid Heart Disease From Primary Ovarian Carcinoid Tumors. Am. J. Med. 45:643, 1968.

Christie, A. C. Three cases Illustrating The Presence Of Argentaffin (Kulchitsky) Cells In The Human Gallbladder. J. Clin. Path. 7:318, 1954.

Christy, N. P. Adrenocorticotrophic Activity In The Plasma Of Patients With Cushing's Syndrome Associated With Pulmonary Neoplasms. Lancet. 1:85, 1961.

Christodoulopoulos, J. B., and Klotz, A. P. Carcinoid Syndrome With Primary Carcinoid Tumor Of The Stomach. Gastroenter. 40:429, 1961.

Churchill, E. D. Discussant in paper by Jackson, C. L. and Kenzelmann, F. W. Bronchoscopic Aspects Of Bronchial Tumors. J. Thor. Surg. 6:335, 1937.

Ciaccio, M. C. Sur Une Nouvelle Espese Cellulaire Dans Les Glandes Der Lieberkuhn. C. R. Soc. Biol. (Paris) 60:76, 1906.

Cohen, R. B., Toll, G. D., and Castleman, B. Bronchial Adenomas In Cushing's Syndrome. Their relation with thymomas and oat cell carcinomas associated with hyperadrenocorticism. Cancer. 13:812, 1960.

Collins, D. C. A Study Of 50,000 Specimens Of The Human Vermiform Appendix. Surg. Gynec. Obstet. 101:437, 1955.

Collins, D. H. and Pugh, R. C. B. Testicular Tumors. Brit. J. Urol. 36:(supplement) 1964.

Cope, Z., and Newcomb, W. D., Metastasis Of An Argentaffin Carcinoma Of The Testicle. Brit. J. Urol. 2:268, 1930.

Cordier, R. Recherches Morphologigues et Experimentates Sur La Cellule Chromoargentaffine de L'epithelium Intestinal des Verte Tres. Arch. Biol. Paris. 36:427, 1926.

Cosh, J., Cates, J. E. and Pugh, D. W. Carcinoid Heart Disease. Brit. Heart. J. 30:491, 1959.

Costello, and Aitken, L. F., Carcinoid Of The Duodenum. Mo. Med. 57:1252, 1960.

Currens, J. H., Kinney, T. D., and White, P. D. Pulmonary Stenosis With Intact Interventricular Septum. Report of eleven cases. Amer. Heart J. 30:491, 1945.

Dalgliesh, C. E. Two Dimensional Paper Chromatography Of Urinary Indoles And Related Substances. Biochem. J. 64:491, 1956.

Danisch, B. Zur Histogenese Der Sog Appendix Carcinoide. Zieglers Beitrage. 122:687, 1924.

Davies, A. J. Carcinoid Tumours (Argentaffinomata) Ann. R. Coll. Surg. Engl. 25:277, 1959.

Davis, R. B. The Concentration Of Serotonin In Normal Human Sera As Determined By An Improved Method. J. Lab. Clin. Med. 54:344, 1959.

Dengler, H. Studies On The Effects Of Synthetic Hypertensin II On Electrolyte Metabolism, Kidney Function And Circulation In Man. Kln. Wschr. 37:1245, 1959.

Devitt, P. G. Carcinoid Tumour Of The Breast. Brit. Med. J. 2:327, 1978.

Dockerty, M. B. and Ashburn, F. S. Carcinoid Tumors Of Ileum: Report of 13 cases in which there were metastasis. Arch. Surg. 47:221, 1943.

Dockerty, M. B. and Sheifley, C. H. Metastasizing Carcinoid: Report of an unusual case with episodic cyanosis. Am. J. Clin. Pathol. 25:770, 1955.

Dockerty, M. B. Carcinoid Tumors. Calif. Med. 99:157, 1963.

Dolezel, S., Filkuka, J., Tomasek, V., and Vlasin, Z. Histochemical Demonstration Of 5-hydroxytryptamine In A Malignant Carcinoid Of The Small Intestine. Neoplasma. 16:209, 1969.

Dollinger, M. R. and Gardner, B. Newer Aspects Of The Carcinoid Spectrum. Surg. Gynec. Obst. 122:1335, 1966.

Dollinger, M. R., Ratner, L. H., Shamoian, C. A., and Blackbourne, B. D. Carcinoid Syndrome Associated With Pancreatic Tumor. Arch. Int. Med. 120:575, 1967.

Douchette, J. W. and Estes, W. B. Primary Ovarian Carcinoid Tumor. Obstet. and Gynec. 25:94, 1965.

Drichman, A. and Hodges, J. H. Carcinoid Of Meckel's Diverticulum. Report Of A Case And Review Of The Literature. Arch. Pathol. 69:701, 1960.

Eklöf, O. Carcinoid Tumors Of The Stomach. A report of three cases with a review of the literature. Acta. Chir. Scand. 121:118, 1961.

Ellison, E. H. Discussion Of Paper By Oberhelman, H. A., Nelson, T. S., and Dragstedt, L. R. Arch. Surg. 77:414, 1958.

Engelman, K., Lovenberg, W., and Sjoerdsma, A. Inhibition Of Serotonin Synthesis By Parachlorphenylalanine In Patients With The Carcinoid Syndrome. New Eng. Med. J. 277:1103, 1967.

Erspamer, V. and Asero, B. Identification Of Enteramine, The Specific Hormone Of The Enterochromaffin Cell System, As 5-hydroxytryptamine. Nature. 169:800, 1952.

Eros, G. Eine Nerve Dartstellung Methode der Sogennannten "Geller" Argentiffinen Zellen des Magendarmtraktes. Zentrabl. Allg. Pathol. 54:385, 1932.

Escovitz, W. E. and Reingold, I. M. Functioning Malignant Bronchial Carcinoid With Cushing's Syndrome And Recurrent Sinus Arrest. Ann. Int. Med. 54:1248, 1961.

Fabricius, J., Jensen, K., and Poulsen, H. E. Metastasizing Carcinoid. Results of cardiac catheterization and autopsy in a case. Dan. Med. Bull. 5:237, 1958.

Felton, W. L., Liebow, A. A., and Lindskog, G. E. Peripheral And Multiple Bronchial Adenomas. Cancer. 6:555, 1953.

Feyrter, F. Uber das Bronchuscarcinoid. Virchows Arch. Path. Anat. 332:25, 1959.

Field, J. L., Adamson, L. F. and Stockle, H. E. Review Of Carcinoids In Children. Functioning carcinoid in a 15 year old male. Pediatrics. 29:953, 1962.

Fischet E. R. and Hicks, J. Further Pathologic Observations On The Syndrome Of Peptic Ulcer And Multiple Endocrine Tumors. Gastroenterol. 38:458, 1960.

Fischer, S. and Lindeneg, O. Cardiac Changes In Argentaffinomatosis. Acta. Path. and Microbiol. Scand. 44:128, 1958.

Forbus, W. D. Argentaffin Tumors Of The Appendix And Small Intestine. Bull. Johns Hopkins Hosp. 37:130, 1925.

Foster-Carter, A. F. Bronchial Adenoma. Quart. J. Med. 10:139, 1941.

Foy, J. M. and Parratt, R. A Note On The Presence Of Noradrenaline And 5-hydroxytryptamine In Plantain. J. Pharm. Pharmocol. 12:360, 1960.

Frantz, V. K. Tumors Of The Pancreas. Armed Forces Inst. Pathol. 27:27, 1959.

Freund, S. J. Carcinoid Tumors Of The Rectum. Am. J. Surg. 93:67, 1957.

Gerber, B. C. and Shields, T. W. Simultaneous Duodenal Carcinoid And Non-beta Cell Tumors Of The Pancreas. Arch. Surg. 81:379, 1960.

Gibbs, N. M. The Histogenesis Of Carcinoid Tumours Of The Rectum. J. Clin. Path. 16:206, 1963.

Gillman, J. A Postmortem Study Of Gastric Argentaffin Cells. S. Afr. Med. J. 7:144, 1942.

Gmelich, J. T., Bensch, K. G., and Liebow, A. A. Cells Of Kulchitsky Type In Bronchioles And Their Relation To Origin Of Peripheral Carcinoid Tumors. Lab. Invest. 17:88, 1967.

Goldman, A. The Malignant Nature Of Bronchial Adenoma. J. Thoracic Surg. 18:137, 1949.

Goldman, N. C., Hood, I. and Singleton, G. T. Carcinoid Of The Larynx. Arch. Otolaryng. 90:90, 1969.

Goodner, J. T., Berg. J. W. and Watson, W. L. The Non-benign Nature Of Bronchial Carcinoids And Cylindromas. Cancer. 14:539, 1961.

Gosset, A. and Masson, P. Tumeurs Endocrines de l'appendize. Presse Med. 22:237, 1914.

Grahame-Smith, D. G. The carcinoid Syndrome. Amer. J. Cardiol. 21:376, 1968.

Greenbaum, D. Multiple Familial Parathyroid Adenomata. Proc. Roy. Soc. Med. 53:903, 1960.

Hale, J. F. and Lane-Mitchell, W. Carcinoid Syndrome. Report of a case with review of the leterature. Central Afr. J. Med. 10:162, 1964.

Hallwright, G. P. and North, K. A. K. Pigmentation And Cushing's Syndrome Due To Malignant Tumor Of The Pancreas. J. Clin. Endocr. 24:496, 1964.

Hamlin, K. E. and Fischer, F. E. The Synthesis Of 5-hydroxytryptamine. J. Am. Chem. Soc. 73:5007, 1951.

Hamperl, H. Uber Gutartiga Bronchial Tumores. Vitchows Arch. Path. Anat. 300:46, 1937.

Hanna, S. M. Carcinoid Syndrome Associated With Psychosis. Postgrad. Med. J. 41:566, 1965.

Hasegawa, V. Ueberdie Carcinoide Der Wurmforsatz. Virchows Arch. 1:294, 1923.

Hawley, P. R. A Case Of Secondary Carcinoid Tumors In Both Breasts, Following Excision Of Primary Carcinoid Tumours Of The Duodenum. Br. J. Surg. 53:818, 1966.

Heine, J. Ueber Eine Primate Gestielle Bronchialgeschwulst. Verhandl des deutscher pathol. Gesell. 22:293, 1927.

Heidenhain, R. Untersuchungen Uber den Bau der Labdrusen. Arch. Mikros Anat. 6:368, 1870.

Hernandez, F. J. and Reid, J. D. Mixed Carcinoid And Mucous-secreting Intestinal Tumors. Arch. Pathol. 88:489, 1969.

Hillman, S. Tricuspid Stenosis And Pulmonary Stenosis Complicating Carcinoid Of Intestine With Metastasis To Liver. Amer. Heart J. 25:391, 1943.

Hilton, S. M. and Lewis, G. P. The Relationship Between Glandular Activity, Bradykinin Formation, And Functional Vasodilatation In The Submaxillary Salivary Gland. J. Physiol. (London) 134:471, 1956.

Holl-Allen, R. T. J. Metastatic Ovarian Carcinoid. Postgrad. Med. J. 45:46, 1969.

Carcinoid Tumors

Holley, S. W. Bronchial Adenoma. Milit. Surg. 99:528, 1946.

Horn, R. C. Carcinoid Tumors Of The Colon And Rectum. Cancer. 2:819, 1949.

House, H. C. and Herman, R. E. Functioning Malignant Carcinoid. A review of nine cases. Clev. Clin. Quart. 32:217, 1965.

Huebschmann, P. Sur Le Carcinome Primitis de L'appendice Vermiculare. Rev. Med. Suisse Romande. 30:317, 1910.

Isler, P. and Hedinger, C. Metastasierendes Dunndarmcarcinoid Mitschweren Vorwiegend das Rechte Herz Betreffenden Klapenfehlern Und Pulmonalstenose-ein Eigenartiger Symptomenkomplex. Schweiz Med. Wochenscht. 83:4, 1953.

Jackson, A. S. Carcinoma Of The Appendix. Arch. Surg. 6:653, 1923.

Jacobson, W. The Argentiffine Cells And Pernicious Anemia. J. Pathol. Bact. 49:1, 1939.

Jacobson, W. and Simpson, D. M. The Fluoresence Spectra Of Pterins And Their Possible Use In The Elucidation Of Antipernicious Factor. Biochem. J. 40:9, 1946.

Janeway, T. C., Richardson, H. B. and Paru, E. A. Experiments On The Vasoconstrictor Action Of Blood Serum. Arch. Int. Med. 21:575, 1918.

Joel, W. Katzinoid der Gallenblase. Zentralbl. Allg. Pathol. 46:1, 1929.

Johnston, R. H., Hall, R. A. and Erikson, E. E. Argentaffin Cell Tumor Of Meckel's Diverticulum. Associated with gastrointestinal bleeding. Arch. Surg. 90:172, 1965.

Kantor, S., Crane, R. D. and Gillesby, W. J. Carcinoid Tumors Of The Gastrointestinal Tract. Am. Surg. 27:448, 1961.

Kaplan, E. L., Sizemore, G. W., Peskin, G. W. and Jaffe, B. M. Humoral Similarities Of Carcinoid Tumors And Medullary Carcinomas Of The Thyroid. Surgery. 74:21, 1973.

Kemble, J. V. H. Argentaffin Carcinomata Of The Testicle. Brit. Urel. 40:580, 1968.

Kinley, C. E. and Penner, D. W. Carcinoid Tumors. A review and clinicopathologic study of 52 cases. Can. J. Surg. 5:138, 1962.

Kowlessar, O. D., Williams, R. C., Law, D. H. and Sleisenger, M. H. Urinary Excretion Of 5-hydroxyindoleacetic Acid In Diarrheal States With Special Reference To Nontropical Sprue. N. Eng. J. Med. 259:340, 1958.

Knowles, C. H. R., McCrea, A. N. and Davis, A. Metastasis From Argentaffinoma Of The Appendix. J. Pathol. Bact. 72:326, 1956.

Kramer, R. Adenoma Of Bronchus. Ann. Otol. Rhin. Laryng. 39:689, 1930.

Krompecher, E. Ueber die Basalzellentumoren der Zylinderepithelsch Eimhante mit Besonderer Berucksichtigung des Katzinoide des Darmes. Beitr. Pathol. Anat. 65:79, 1919.

Kulchitsky, N. Zur Stage Ueber den bau des Darmkanals. Arch. F. Mikr. Anat. 49:7, 1899.

Langhans, T. Ueber Einen Drusenpolyp Im Ileum. Virchows Arch. Pathol. Anat. 38:559, 1867.

Latham, W. D., Arnold, H. S. and Ede, S. Kulchitsky-cell Carcinoma (carcinoid) Of The Appendix With Metastasis. Am. J. Surg. 102:607, 1961.

Lattes, R. and Grossi. Carcinoid Tumors Of The Stomach. Cancer. 9:698, 1956.

Lechner, G. W. and Chamblin, S. A., Jr. Carcinoid Tumors Of Meckel's Diverticula. Am. J. Surg. 103:166, 1962.

Legha, S. S., Valdevieso, M., Nelson, R. R., Benjamin, R. S. and Bodey, G. P. Chemotherapy For Metastatic Carcinoid Tumors. Experience with 32 patients and a review of the literature. Cancer Treatment Reports. 61:1699, 1977.

Lembeck, F. 5-hydroxytryptamine In A Carcinoid Tumour. Nature. 172:910, 1953.

Levine, R. J. and Sjoerdsma, A. Pressor Amines And The Carcinoid Flush. Ann. Int. Med. 58:818, 1963.

Liebow, A. A. Tumor Of The Lower Respiratory Tract. In Atlas Of Tumor Pathology. Sect. 5. Fasc. 17. 1952. Armed Forces Inst. Path. Washington, D.C.

Lillie, R. D. and Glenner, G. G. Carcinoid Tumors Of The Human Gastrointestinal Tract. Am. J. Pathol. 36:623, 1960.

Lillie, R. D., Greco-Henson, J. P. and Cason, J. P. Azo-coupling Rate Of Enterochromaffin With Various Diazonium Salts. J. Histochem. Cytochem. 9:11, 1961.

Lubarsch, O. Ueber den Primaren Krebs des Ileum Nebst Bemerkungen Ueber das Gleichzeitige Vorkommen Von Krebs Und Tuberculose. Virchows Arch. Pathol. Anat. 111:280, 1888.

Ludwig, C. and Schmidt, A. Das Verhalten der Gase, Welche mit dem Blut Durch den Reizbaren Saügtethiermuskel Stromen. Arb. Physiol. Anstalt. Z. Leipzig 3: Fasc. 12.1, 1868.

Ludwig, G. D., Cushard, W., Bartuska, D., Franco, R. and Chaykin, L. Effects Of Beta-adrenergic Blockade In The Carcinoid Syndrome. Ann. Int. Med. 68:1188, 1968.

McDonald, R. A. A study Of 356 Carcinoids Of The Gastrointestinal Tract. Report of four new cases of the carcinoid syndrome. Amer. J. Med. 21:867, 1956.

McDonald R. A., Robbins, S. L. and Mallory, G. K. Morphologic Effects Of Serotonin (5-hydroxytryptamine). Arch. Path. 65:369, 1958.

Mattingly, T. W. and Sjoerdsma, A. The Cardiovascular Manifestations Of Functioning Carcinoid Tumors. Mod. Concepts Cardiovasc. Dis. 25:337, 1956.

Markgraf, W. H. and Dunn, T. M. Appendiceal Carcinoid With Carcinoid Syndrome. Am. J. Surg. 107:730, 1964.

Marshall, A. H. E. and Sloper, J. C. Pluriglandular Adenomatosis Of The Pituitary, Parathyroid And Pancreatic-islet Cells Associated With Lipomatosis. J. Path. Bact. 68:225, 1954.

Masson, P. Carcinoids (Argentaffin Cell Tumors) And Nerve Hyperplasia Of Appendicular Mucosa. Am. J. Path. 4:181, 1928.

McCartney, E. T. and Stewart, I. Argentaffin Tumor Of The Ileum With Intussusception. Br. Med. J. 1:769, 1959.

McCracken, J. D. and Davenport. O. L. Carcinoid Of The Stomach With Giant Duodenal Ulcer. Am. J. Surg. 110:776, 1965.

McKusick, V. A. Carcinoid Cardiovascular Disease. Bull. Johns Hopkins Hosp. 98:13, 1956.

McMullen, F. F. and Hanson, H. H. Carcinoid Syndrome In Pancreatic Carcinoma. Circulation. 18:883, 1958.

Melmon, K. L., Sjoerdsma, A., Oates, J. A. and Laster, L. Treatment Of Malabsorption And Diarrhea Of The Carcinoid Syndrome With Methysergide. Gastroenter. 48:18, 1963.

Melmon, K. L., Lovenberg, W. and Sjoerdsma, A. Identification Of Lysyl-bradykinin As The Peptide Formed In Vitro By Carcinoid Tumor Kallikrein. Clin. Chim. Acta. 12:292, 1965.

Mengel, C. E. Cutaneous Manifestations Of The Malignant Carcinoid Syndrome. Ann. Int. Med. 58:989, 1963.

Mengel, C. E. Therapy Of Malignant Carcinoid Syndrome. Ann. Int. Med. 62:587, 1965.

Merling. F. Anatomic Pathologique de L'appendice du Caecum. Experience (Paris) 1:337, 1838.

Moersch, H. J. and McDonald, J. R. Bronchial Adenoma. J. Am. Med. Assoc. 142:299, 1950.

Moertel, C. G., Sauer, W. G., Dockerty, M. B. and Baggensoss. Life History Of The Carcinoid Tumor Of The Small Intestine. Cancer. 14:901, 1961.

Moertel, C. G., Beahrs, O. H., Woolner, L. B. and Tyce, G. M. "Malignant Carcinoid Syndrome" Associated With Non-carcinoid Tumor. New Eng. J. Med. 273:244, 1965.

Moertel, C. G., Dockerty, M. B. and Judd, E. S. Carcinoid Tumors Of The Vermiform Appendix. Cancer. 15:270, 1967.

Moertel, C. G. Reitemeier, R. J. and Schutt, A. J. Phase II Study Of Streptozotocin In The Treatment Of Advanced Gastrointestinal Cancer. Cancer Chemother. Rep. 55:303, 1971.

Morgan, J. G., Marks, C. and Hearn, C. D. Carcinoid Tumors Of The Gastrointestinal Tract. Ann. Surg. 180:720, 1974.

Morson, B. S. In Modern Trends In Gastroenterology. Edited by F. Avery-Jones. London. Butterworth.

Mueller, H. Zut Entschungsgeschichte des Bronchialer Weiterungen. Inaug. Diss. Halle. 1882.

Murray-Lyon, I. M., Dawson, J. L., Rake, M. D. Blendis, L. M., Laws, J. W. and Williams, R. Treatment Of Secondary Hepatic Tumors By Ligation Drugs. Abstr. Brit. Soc. Of Gastroenterol. Gut. 10:1057, 1969.

Naclerio, E. A. and Langer, L. Adenoma Of The Bronchus. Am. J. Surg. 75:532, 1948.

Nance, F. C. and Thomas, M. A. Diagnosis And Treatment Of The Zollinger-Ellison Syndrome. J. Louisiana Med. Soc. 120:91, 1968.

Nash, D. T. and Brin, M. Malabsorption In Malignant Carcinoid With Normal 5-HIAA. New York J. Med. 64:1128, 1964.

Notthaft. A. Ueber Einem Fall Multiplier Primärkrebse Des Dünndarmes. Deutsch. Med. Wchnscht. 14:691, 1896.

Nunes, W. P. Unusual Case Of Carcinoid Of The Stomach With Clinical And X-ray Symptoms Of Cardial Stenosis. Rev. Assoc. Med. Bras. 4:37–42, 1958.

Oates, J. A., Melmon, K., Sjoerdsma, A. Gillespie, L. and Mason, D. T. Release Of A Kinin Peptide In The Carcinoid Syndrome. Lancet 1:514, 1964.

Oates, J. A. and Butler, T. C. Pharmacoligic And Endocrine Aspects Of Carcinoid Syndrome. Adv. Pharmacol. 5:109, 1967.

Oberndorfer, S. Ueber die Kleinen Dunndarmcarcinome. Verh. Dtsch. Ges. Pathol. 11:113, 1907.

Orloff, M. J. Carcinoid Tumors Of The Rectum. Cancer. 28:175, 1971.

Pack, G. T. Unusual Tumors Of The Stomach. Ann. N. Y. Acad. Sc. 114:985, 1964.

Page, I. H. Serotonin (5-hydroxytryptamine). The Last Four Years. Physiol. Rev. 38:277, 1958.

Page, I. H. and McCubbin, J. W. The Variable Arterial Pressure Response To Serotonin In Laboratory Animals And Man. Circ. Res. 1:354, 1953.

Paneth, J. Ueber die Secernirenden Zellen des Dunndarm-Epithels. Arch. F. Mikr. Anat. 31:113, 1888.

Parat, M. Histophysiology Of Digestive Organs In Embryo. Compt. Rend. Soc. de Biol. 90:1023, 1924.

Pataky, Y., Nagi, L. and Popik, E. Uber Einen Nom Pancreaskoft Hervorgehenden Primaren Argentaffin Tumorfall. Zbl. Allg. Path. (Jena). 99:442, 1959.

Pearson, C. M. and Fitzgerald, P. J. Carcinoid Tumors—A Reemphasis Of Their Malignant Nature. Review of 140 cases. Cancer. 2:1005, 1949.

Peart, W. S. and Robertson, J. I. S. The Effect Of A Serotonin Antagonist (UML 491) In Carcinoid Disease. Lancet 2:1172, 1961.

Peart, W. S., Porter, K. A., Robertson, J. I. S., Sandler, M. and Baldock, E. Carcinoid Syndrome Due To Pancreatic-duct Neoplasm Secreting 5-hydroxytryptophan and 5-hydroxytryptamine. Lancet. 1:239, 1963.

Peart, W. S. Carcinoid Tumors. Acta. Med. Scand. (Suppl.) 179:445, 1966.

Pernow, B. and Waldenstrom, J. Determination Of 5-hydroxytryptamine, 5-hydroxyindoleacetic Acid And Histamine In 33 Cases Of Carcinoid Tumors. Am. J. Med. 23:16, 1957.

Perlman, R. M. Pluriglandular Adenomatosis. Arch. Path. 38:20, 1944.

Persaud, V. and Walrond, E. R. Carcinoid Tumor And Cystadenoma Of The Pancreas. Arch. Path. 92:28, 1971.

Peskin, G. W. and Orloff, M. J. A Clinical Study Of 25 Patients With Carcinoid Tumors Of The Rectum. Surg. Gynec. Obstet. 109:673, 1959.

Pestana, C., Beahts, O. H. and Woolner, L. B. Multiple (seven) Carcinoids Of The Stomach. Proc. Mayo Clin. 38:453, 1963.

Pollard, A., Grainger, R. G. and Fleming, O. An Unusual Case Of Metastasizing Bronchial "Adenoma" Associated With The Carcinoid Syndrome. Lancet. 2:1084, 1962.

Ponka, J. L. and Antoni, R. O. Surgical Management Of Appendiceal Carcinoids. Henry Ford Hosp. Med. Bull. 11:431, 1963.

Postlethwait, R. W. Gastrointestinal Carcinoid Tumors. Postgrad. Med. 40:455, 1966.

Price-Thomas, C. Benign Tumours Of The Lung. Lancet. 1:2, 1954.

Prunty, F. T. G. and Smith, P. M. Successful Treatment Of Cushing's Syndrome Secondary To An Argentaffinoma By Bilateral Adrenalectomy. Proc. Royal Soc. Med. 58:573, 1965.

Raboni, F. and Maestri, A. Sul Carcinoide O Argentaffinoma Dello Stomaco. Giorn. Clin. Med. 42:1313, 1961.

Ransom, W. B. A Case Of Primary Carcinoma Of The Ileum. Lancet. 2:1020: 1890.

Rapport, M. M., Green, A. A. and Page, I. H. Partial Purification Of The Vasoconstrictor In Bees Serum. J. Biol. Chem. 174:735, 1948.

Reid, D. R. K. Argentaffinoma Of The Gastrointestinal Tract. Br. J. Surg. 36:130, 1948.

Reid, J. D. Adenoid Cystic Carcinoma Of Bronchial Tree. Cancer 5:685, 1952.

Reddy, D. V., Adams, F. H. and Baird, C. Teratogenic Effects Of Serotonin. J. Pediatrics 63:394, 1963.

Reingold, I. M. and Escovitz, W. E. Metastatic Cutaneous Carcinoid. Report of a case of functioning malignant bronchial carcinoid. Arch. Dermatol. 82:971, 1960.

Reisner, D. Intrabronchial Polypoid Adenoma. Arch. Surg. 16:1201, 1928.

Reuter, S. R. and Boijsen, E. Angiographic Findings In Two Ileal Carcinoid Tumors. Radiology 87:836, 1966.

River, L., Silverstein, J. and Tope, J. W. Benign Neoplasms Of The

Small Intestine. A critical comprehensive review with report of 20 new cases. Int. Abstr. Surg. 102:1, 1956.

Roberts, W. C. and Sjoerdsma, A. The Cardiac Disease Associated With The Carcinoid Syndrome (carcinoid heart disease). Am. J. Med. 36:5, 1964.

Robertson, J. I. S., Peart, W. S. and Andrews T. M. The Mechanism Of Facial Flush In The Carcinoid Syndrome. Quart. J. Med. 31:103, 1962.

Rocklin, D. B. and Longmire, W. P. Jr. Primary Tumors Of The Small Intestine. Surgery 50:586, 1961.

Rosenbaum, F. F., Santer, D. G. and Claudon, D. B. Essential Telangiectasia Pulmonic And Tricuspid Stenosis, And Neoplastic Liver Disease. A possible new clinical syndrome. J. Lab. Clin. Med. 42:941, 1953.

Roth, M. Carcinoid Of The Rectum. A case report with observations on radiosensitivity of nodular metastases to the skin. Am. J. Roentgenol. 86:97, 1961.

Saegesser, F. and Gross, M. Carcinoid Syndrome And Carcinoid Tumors Of The Rectum. Am. J. Proctol. 20:27, 1969.

Saltykow, S. Uber Die Genese der "Karzinoiden Tumoren" Sowie der "Adenomyome" des Darmes. Beitr. Z. Pathol. Anat. 54:559, 1912.

Souders, C. R. and Kingsley, J. W. Bronchial Adenoma. New Eng. J. Med. 239:459, 1948.

Sandler, M. and Snow, P. J. D. An Atypical Carcinoid Tumour Secreting 5-hydroxytryptophan. Lancet. 1:137, 1958.

Sauer, W. G., Dearing, W. H., Flock, E. V., Waugh, J. M., Dockerty, M. B. and Roth, G. M. Functioning Carcinoid Tumors. Gastroenterol. 34:216, 1958.

Schneckloth, R. E., Page, I. H., Del Greco, F. and Corcoran, A. C. Effects Of Serotonin Antagonists In Normal Subjects And Patients With Carcinoid Tumors. Circulation 16:523, 1957.

Schneckloth, R. E., McIsaac, W. M. and Page, I. H. Serotonic Metabolism In Carcinoid Syndrome With Metastatic Bronchial Adenoma. J.A.M.A. 170, 1959.

Schwandt, R. Kasvisticher Beitrag Zum Karzinoid des Magens. Z. Gesamte Inn. Med. 16:388, 1961.

Scully, R. E. Recent Progress In Ovarian Cancer. Human Pathol. 1:73, 1970.

Sethl, G. and Hardin, C. E. Primary Malignant Tumors Of The Small Bowel. Arch. Surg. 98:659, 1969.

Shames, J. M., Dhurandhat, N. R. and Blackard, W. G. Insulin-secreting Bronchial Carcinoid Tumor With Widespread Metastases. Amer. J. Med. 44:632, 1968.

Shorb, P. E. Jr. and McCune, W. S. Carcinoid Tumors Of The Gastro-intestinal Tract. An analysis of 70 cases. Am. J. Surg. 107:329, 1964.

Simon, H. B., McDonald, J. R. and Culp, C. S. Argentaffin Tumor (carcinoid) Occurring In A Benign Cystic Teratoma Of The Testicle. J. Urol. 72:892, 1954.

Sinnetamby, R. C., Gordon, A. B. and Griffith, J. D. The Occurrence Of Carcinoid Tumor In Teratoma Of The Testis. Brit. J. Surg. 60:576, 1973.

Sjoerdsma, A., Weissbach, H. and Udenfriend, S. Simple Test For Diagnosis Of Metastatic Carcinoid (argentaffinoma). J.A.M.A. 159:397, 1955.

Sjoerdsma, A., Weissbach, H., Terry, L. L. and Udenfriend, S. Further Observations On Patients With Malignant Carcinoid. Am. J. Med. 23:5, 1957.

Sjoerdsma, A., Oates, J. A. Zaltman, P. and Udenfriend, S. Serotonin Synthesis In Carcinoid Patients: It's Inhibition By X-methyl-dopa With Measurement Of Associated Increase In Urinary 5-hydroxytryptophan. New Eng. J. Med. 263:585, 1960.

Southern, A. L. Functioning Metastatic Bronchial Carcinoid With Elevated Levels Of Serum And Cerebrospinal Fluid Serotonin And Pituitary Adenoma. J. Clin. Endoct. 20:298, 1960.

Stewart, M. J. and Taylor, A. L. Carcinoid Tumor Of Meckel's Diverticulum. J. Pathol. Bact. 29:135, 1926.

Stewart, M. J., Willis, R. A. and De Saram, G. S. W. Argentaffine Carcinoma In Terratoma. J. Path. Bact. 49:207, 1939.

Thomas, B. M. Three Unusual Carcinoid Tumors With Particular Reference To Osteoblastic Bone Metastases. Clin. Radiol. 19:221, 1968.

Thompson, N. W. and Coon, W. W. Carcinoid Of The Stomach. Am. J. Surg. 108:798, 1964.

Thorson, A., Bjorck, G., Bjorkman, G. and Waldenstrom, J. Malignant Carcinoid Of The Small Intestine With Metastases To The Liver, Valvular Disease Of The Right Side Of The Heart;

Bronchoconstriction And An Unusual Type Of Cyanosis. A clinicopathologic syndrome. Am. Heart J. 47:795, 1954.

Thorson, A. Studies On Carcinoid Disease. Acta Med. Scand. (suppl.) 334:1, 1958.

Thorson, A., Hanson, A., Pernow, B., Söderström, J., Winblad, S. and Wulff, H. B. Carcinoid Tumor Within An Ovarian Teratoma In A Patient With The Carcinoid Syndrome. Acta. Med. Scand. 161:495, 1958.

Toenniessen, E. Untersuchungen Uber Die In Der Submukosa Des Dunndarms Vorkommenden Epitheliaten Tumoren. Z. Krebf-forch. 8:355, 1910.

Toker, C. Ovarian Carcinoid. A light and electronmicroscopic study. Am. J. Obstet. Gynecol. 103:1019, 1969.

Toomey, F. B. and Felson, B. Osteoblastic Bone Metastasis In Gastro-intestinal And Bronchial Carcinoids. Am. J. Roentgenol. 83:709, 1960.

Törö, E. Uber Enterochromaffine Zellen. Verh. d. Anat. Gesellsch. 38:49, 1929.

Torvik, A. Carcinoid Syndrome In A Primary Tumor Of The Ovary. Acta Pathol. Microbiol. Scand. 48:81, 1960.

Trappe, M. Ueber Geschwulstartige Fehlbildungen Von Niere, Milz, Haut und Darm. Frankf. Ztschr. F. Pathol. 1:109, 1907.

Trevenen, C., Banerjee, R. and Laughlan, S. C. Primary Carcinoids Of The Ovary. Cancer 31:1482, 1973.

Udenfriend, S., Weissbach, H. and Clark, C. P. The Estimation Of 5-hydroxytryptamine (serotonin) In Biological Tissues. J. Biol. Chem. 215:337, 1955.

Underdahl, L. O., Woolner, L. B. and Black, B. M. Multiple Endo-crine Adenomas: Report of 8 cases in which the parathyroid, pituitary and pancreatic islets were involved. J. Clin. Endocr. 13:20, 1953.

Vaeth, J. M., Rousseau, R. E. and Purcell, T. R. Radiation Response Of Carcinoid Of The Rectum. Am. J. Roentgenol Radium Ther. Nucl. Med. 88:967, 1962.

Van Der Sluys Veer, J., Choufoer, J. C., Querido, A., Van der Heul, R. O., Hollander, C. F. and Van Rijssel, T. G. Metastasizing Islet-cell Tumour Of The Pancreas Associated With Hypogly-cemia And Carcinoid Syndrome. Lancet. 1:1416, 1964.

Vajda, D. and Zulik, R. Magenkarzinoid. Fortschr. Roentgenstr. 96:566, 1962.

Von Bernheimer, H., Ehringer, H., Heistrachet, P., Kraupp, O., Lachnit, V., Obiditsch Mayer, I. and Wenz, M. Biologically Active Non-metastasizing Carcinoid Of The Bronchus With The Left Heart Syndrome. Wein Klin. Wochenschr. 72:867, 1960.

Vyborny, J., Poncarova, Z. and Schlupek, A. Karcinoid Zaludku. Rozhl. Chir. 38:279, 1960.

Waldenström, J., and Ljungberg, E. Case Of Metastasizing Carcinoma Of Unknown Origin Showing Peculiar Flushing And Increased Amounts Of Histamine And 5-hydroxytryptamine In Blood And Urine. Acta. Med. Scand. 153:73, 1956.

Waldenstrom, J. Clinico-pathologic Findings In Carcinoid Heart Disease. Am. J. Med. 54:433, 1973.

Warner, R. R. P., Kirschner, P. A. and Warner, G. M. Serotonin Production By Bronchial Adenoma Without The Carcinoid Syndrome. J.A.M.A. 178:1175, 1961.

Watkins, E. Jr., Khazei, A. M. and Nahra, S. Surgical Basis For Arterial Infusion Chemotherapy Of Disseminated Carcinoma Of The Liver. Surg. Gynecol. Obstet. 130:581, 1970.

Warren, K. W. and Coyle, E. B. Carcinoid Tumors Of The Gastrointestinal Tract. Am. J. Surg. 82:372, 1951.

Waugh, J. M. and Snyder, J. M. Carcinoid Tumor Of The Cecum. Ann. Surg. 114:151, 1941.

Weichert, R. F., Reed, Rand Creech O. Jr. Carcinoid-islet Cell Tumors Of The Duodenum. Ann. Surg. 165:660, 1967.

Weichert, R. F., Roth, L. M., Krementz, E. T., Hewitt, R. L. and Drapanas, T. Carcinoid Islet Cell Tumors Of The Duodenum. Am. J. Surg. 121:195, 1971.

Weisburg, F. and Schaefer, G. L. Carcinoid Tumors And Glycogenolysis. Am. J. Clin. Path. 22:1169, 1952.

Weiss, L. and Ingram, M. Adenomatoid Bronchial Tumors. Two major independent types. Cancer. 14:161, 1961.

Wermer, P. Genetic Aspects Of Adenomatosis Of Endocrine Glands. Amer. J. Med. 16:363, 1954.

Williams, E. D. and Azzopardi, J. G. Tumors Of The Lung And The Carcinoid Syndrome. Thorax. 15:30, 1960.

Williams, E. D. and Celestin, L. R. The Association Of Bronchial Carcinoid And Pluriglandular Adenomatosis. Thorax. 17:20, 1962.

Williams, E. D. and Sandler, M. The Classification Of Carcinoid Tumors. Lancet. 1:238, 1963.

Williams, R. A. Metastasizing Carcinoid Tumor With Unusual Features. Brit. Med. J. 1:28, 1960.

Willis, R. A. Argentaffin Carcinomata ("carcinoids") Of The Small Intestine. Med. J. Aust. 2:400, 1940.

Wilson, H. and Butterick, O. D. Massive Liver Resection For Control Of Severe Vasomotor Reactions Secondary To Malignant Carcinoid. Ann. Surg. 149:641, 1959.

Wilson, H., Storer, E. H. and Star, F. J. Carcinoid Tumors. A study of 78 cases. Am. J. Surg. 105:35, 1963.

Willox, S. W. Carcinoid Tumors Of The Appendix In Childhood. Brit. J. Surg. 51:110, 1964.

Womack, N. A. and Graham, E. A. Mixed Tumors Of The Lung, So Called Bronchial Or Pulmonary Adenoma. Arch. Path. 26:165, 1938.

Wu, C. K. Gastric Carcinoid. Zhong Fang Zazhi (Peking) 7:286, 1959.

Zakharia, A. T. Rectal Carcinoids. A review of the literature and report of three new cases. Arch. Surg. 98:8, 1969.

Zarafonetis, C. J. D., Lorber, S. H. and Hanson, S. M. Association Of Functioning Carcinoid Syndrome And Scleroderma. Am. J. Med. Sci. 236:1, 1958.

Zellos, S. Bronchial Adenoma. A study of 40 cases. Thorax. 17:61, 1962.

Zollinger, R. M. and Ellison, E. H. Primary Peptic Ulceration Of The Jejunum With Islet Cell Tumors Of The Pancreas. Ann. Surg. 142:709, 1955.

Index

Index

Index

Pilocarpine, 12
Pituitary, 10
Platelets, 12, 15
Pluriglandular adenomatosis, 59
Pneumonectomy,43
Pneumonia, 42
Polyendocrine factors, 3, 59
Polyhormonal disorders, 11
Polypeptides, 19
Portal blood levels, 18
Prednisone, 120
Pressor
    amines, 15
    response, 17
Prostaglandin, 73
Pseudopodia, 37
Psychosis, 111
Pulmonary
    stenosis, 13, 101, 109
    effects, 18
Pyridoxine, 117

Radiotherapy, 114
Radioimmunioassay, 20
Rauwolfia drugs, 18
Rectal carcinoids, 26
Rectum, 2, 22, 23, 26, 85
Renal effects, 17
Reserpine, 17, 33
Respiratory effects, 108
Rests, 8
    epithelial, 9
Retroperitoneal fibrosis, 108, 119

Sacrococcygeal, 99
Sansert, 119
Secretin, 13
Serotonin, 10, 12, 14, 17, 57
Serum, 12, 113
Silver
    impregnation, 9
    staining, 8, 33, 34

Sipple's Disease, 11
Small intestine, 73
Sodium, 20
Spectrophotofluorometry, 112
Stomach, 2, 26, 65
Streptozotocin, 116
Surgical extirpation, 114
Sympathetic nerve, 10
Syndrome
    carcinoid, 3, 14, 58, 79, 96,
      101
    polyendocrine, 3, 59
    treatment, 114
    Zollinger-Ellison, 71, 94

Telangiectasis, 105
Teratoma, 21, 97
Testis, 98
Thyroid
    and medullary carcinoma, 11,
      73
Trasylol, 119
Treatment,
    carcinoid syndrome, 114
Tricuspid regurgitation, 13, 101,
      109
Tryptophan, 5, 12, 14, 15, 58
Tuberculosis, 44, 51
Tubular reabsorption, 17

Ultraviolet, 35
Uranyl acetate, 36

Valvular disease, 13, 59, 101, 109
Vasoconstrictor, 12, 17
Vasomotor, 13
Vascular changes, 79

Wheezing, 18, 108

Zollinger-Ellison syndrome, 71,
      94